the wholegrain diet miracle

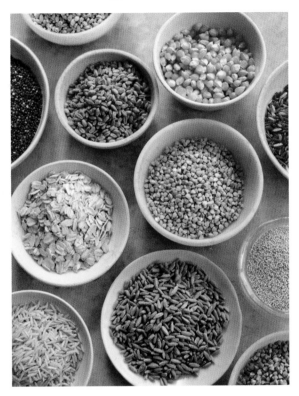

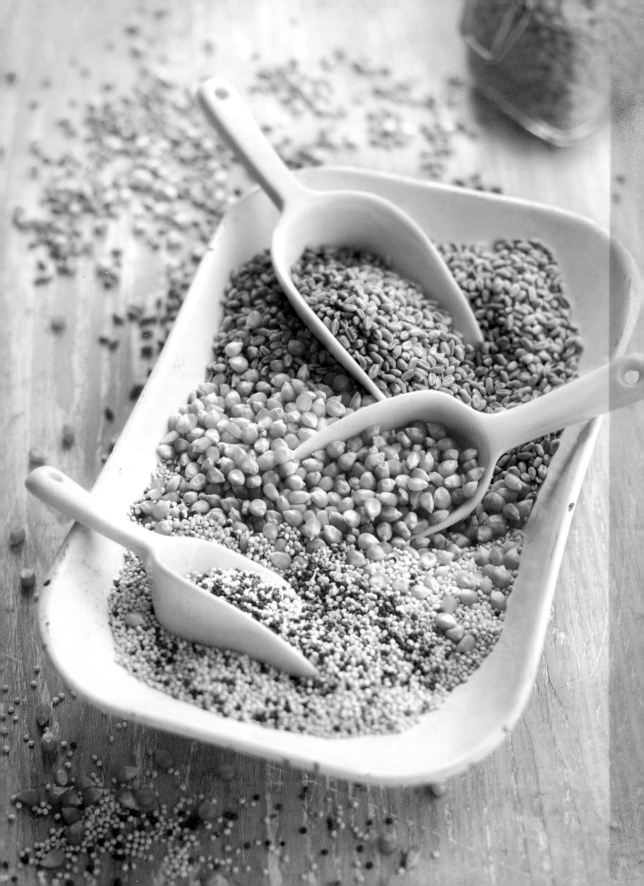

the wholegrain diet miracle

by Dr Lisa Hark & Dr Darwin Deen

DK

LONDON, NEW YORK, MELBOURNE, MUNICH, DELHI

Project editor: Helen Murray
Project designer: Vicky Read
Senior editor: Shannon Beatty
Senior art editor: Anne Fisher
DTP designer: Sonia Charbonnier
Production controllers: Sarah Sherlock, Luca Frassinetti
Photographer: Kate Whitaker
Photography art direction: Luis Peral
Managing editor: Penny Warren
Managing art editor: Marianne Markham
Publishing operations manager: Gillian Roberts
Creative publisher: Mary-Clare Jerram
Art director: Peter Luff
Publishing director: Corinne Roberts

First published in Great Britain in 2006 by Dorling Kindersley Limited,
80 Strand, London WC2R 0RL
Penguin Group (UK)

Copyright © 2006 Dorling Kindersley Limited
Text copyright © 2006 Lisa Hark and Darwin Deen

2 4 6 8 10 9 7 5 3 1

A CIP catalogue record for this book is available from the British Library

ISBN–10: 1–4053–1689–6
ISBN–13: 978–1–4053–1689–7

Colour reproduction by GRB, Italy
Printed and bound by Tien Wah Press, Singapore
Discover more at
www.dk.com

contents

introduction

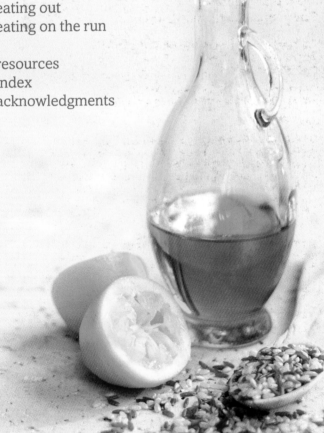

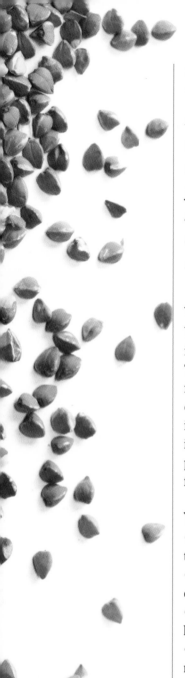

introduction

For the first time in history, we can prescribe a weight-loss diet that has a tremendous amount of scientifically proven health benefits. Eating more wholegrains in their natural form will help you not only to control your weight, but also to reduce your risk of heart disease, diabetes, stroke, and colon cancer, as well as to lower your blood pressure and cholesterol levels. Eating wholegrains has been shown to save lives and reduce death rates. So what are you waiting for? It's easier than you think.

What are wholegrains?

Wholegrains are the form of the grain as it exists in nature. A wholegrain is the entire seed of the plant, consisting of the bran, endosperm, and germ. The bran, or the multilayer outer skin, provides the majority of the grain's fibre, and also B vitamins, minerals, antioxidants, and phytochemicals. The endosperm, or middle layer, is the largest portion of the grain or seed and is the source of protein, carbohydrates, and some vitamins. The germ, or inner layer, is a rich source of vitamins, trace minerals, unsaturated fats, phytochemicals, and antioxidants, which are different from those found in fruits and vegetables and unique to wholegrains.

What are the functions of these vitamins and minerals?

- **Thiamin** (vitamin B_1) helps to convert food into energy, and maintains the proper functioning of the heart, nervous system, and digestive system.
- **Riboflavin** (vitamin B_2) is necessary for the release of energy from carbohydrates, and helps to digest fats and protect the nervous system.
- **Niacin** (vitamin B_3) is involved in energy release from food, and may help to lower high cholesterol.
- **Folate** is a B vitamin that is vital in the formation of red blood cells. It reduces the risk of birth defects and may reduce the risk of heart disease.
- **Iron** is an essential mineral and a component of haemoglobin, which transports oxygen around the body to all cells.
- **Phosphorus** is a mineral that is essential for strong bones and teeth. It is also vital for the production of energy from food.
- **Calcium,** a mineral, is essential for bone strength, and plays an important role in muscle contractions and in normal blood clotting.
- **Magnesium** is a mineral that helps muscles to relax and is vital for a healthy heart and nervous system.

- **Copper,** a mineral, plays a key role in the development of healthy bones, teeth, and heart, and in protecting cells from chemical damage, since it acts as an antioxidant. It is also involved in the formation of red blood cells.
- **Manganese** is a trace mineral that is needed for the body to break down carbohydrates, proteins, and fats. It is also thought to be involved in the balancing of blood sugar levels.
- **Selenium** is an antioxidant that protects cells from the damaging effects of free radicals, which can lead to heart disease. It strengthens the immune system, and is thought to have anti-cancer properties.

A wholegrain is the entire seed of the plant, consisting of the bran, endosperm, and germ.

What are the benefits of antioxidants and phytochemicals?

Antioxidants are substances naturally occurring in foods that help neutralize the damaging effects of free radicals, which occur as by-products of normal metabolic processes. If the body's supply of antioxidants is insufficient, the risk of developing heart disease and cancer can increase. Sources of antioxidants include vitamins A, C, and E, and the minerals copper, selenium, and zinc. Wholegrains contain a variety of unique antioxidants.

Phytochemicals are natural substances produced by plants to protect the plant from viruses and bacteria, and are also believed to benefit the human immune system, defending it against heart disease, cancer, and diabetes. The best way to get phytochemicals in the diet is from natural, unprocessed foods, such as wholegrains, beans, fruits, and vegetables. The bran and germ portions of the wholegrain are a rich source of phytochemicals.

How are grains refined?

Refined grains are stripped of the bran and germ during the milling process – usually to make white flour – leaving only the endosperm portion behind. Without the bran and the germ, there is very little fibre. Refining also reduces the protein content by 25 per cent and removes 17 key nutrients and most of the phytochemicals and antioxidants – all of which make refined products unhealthy choices. However, because refining increases a product's shelf-life, it is favoured by the food industry. Although manufacturers enrich or fortify most refined foods with some missing

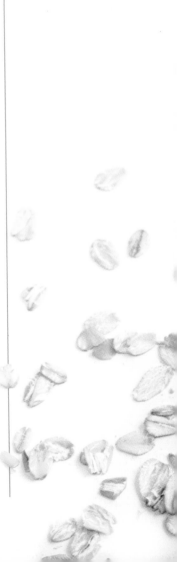

nutrients, fortification does not make up for the vast stores of lost vitamins, minerals, and fibre. In addition, the wholegrain components (germ, endosperm, and bran) seem to work together as a unit; the interplay of healthy nutrients is damaged when they're refined.

Why are wholegrains so good for you?

Wholegrains are a rich source of fibre, vitamins, minerals, antioxidants, and phytochemicals. Over 80 scientific studies have shown that eating more wholegrains can help control your weight and reduce your risk of heart disease, stroke, diabetes, and cancer. These benefits are most likely due to a reduction in blood pressure and cholesterol, as well as a decrease in insulin resistance. Wholegrains help to make you feel full and curb blood sugar spikes that trigger appetite. We describe many of the studies supporting these claims in the Health Benefits section (*see pp10–27*).

Use the recipes and diet plans to help you to eat at least three servings of wholegrains every day.

How much do I need to eat to experience these benefits?

Nutrition experts recommend we eat three to five servings of wholegrains every day. (One serving is 30 grams/1oz or one slice of wholegrain bread). Most of us eat less than one serving of wholegrains daily, or none at all. Use the recipes and diet plans for delicious menu ideas to help you to eat at least three servings of wholegrains every day. We offer advice and tips on undertaking the diet plan and also how to make a gradual transition to wholegrains on pages 66–67.

How can I distinguish between wholegrains and fibre?

Both fibre and wholegrains are healthy but they are not the same. It is important to note that just because a food is high in fibre, it is not necessarily a good source of wholegrains. In fact, wholegrain foods vary in fibre content. Looking at the fibre content alone may not help you to determine whether the food is a good source of wholegrain. For example, wholegrain cereals, such as shredded wheat, have less fibre than bran cereals because bran cereals have the bran (outer hull) of the wheat kernel added in extra amounts (more than was present in the wholegrain).

What is the difference between soluble and insoluble fibre?

Wholegrains are rich in soluble and insoluble fibre, both of which are important for maintaining a healthy digestive system. Soluble fibre, found in oats, barley, and rye, as well as legumes, beans, and citrus fruit, slows the breakdown and absorption of sugar, possibly leading to reduced levels of sugar in the blood. This may explain why there is a reduced risk of developing type 2 diabetes in people who eat wholegrains on a daily basis. During digestion, soluble fibre forms a gel-like substance that binds bile acids, which are needed for cholesterol absorption. If eaten in sufficient quantities, this type of fibre can help reduce the quantity of cholesterol in the blood, which may explain why eating wholegrains reduces the risk of developing heart disease.

Insoluble fibre, found in wholewheat, brown rice, and leafy vegetables, does not dissolve easily in water and is not digested or absorbed by the body. It helps keep the gastrointestinal tract clear and promotes regular bowel movements. Therefore, eating more insoluble fibre may be protective against colon cancer as well as helping to prevent other gastrointestinal disorders (*see pp24–25 for more information*).

Can I still eat wholegrains if I am allergic to gluten?

If your doctor has diagnosed you with coeliac disease or requires you to eliminate gluten from your diet, the grains you should stay away from include all types of wheat (cracked, bulgur, durum, spelt, couscous, kamut, and triticale) as well as oats, rye, and barley. Be careful when inspecting ingredient lists for the presence of gluten: unless a grain product specifically says it is gluten-free, it should be assumed that gluten is present. Depending on your symptoms, it may be necessary to eliminate completely or just partially eliminate these specific grains from your diet. Talk to your doctor about your specific dietary needs. There is no reason to eliminate all wholegrains even if you have a gluten allergy, because there are many nutrient-dense, high-fibre wholegrains that are naturally gluten-free such as rice, buckwheat, amaranth, corn, and quinoa.

Your complete wholegrain handbook

In this book we provide you with advice on buying, storing, cooking, and eating wholegrains. We describe common grains (barley, buckwheat, corn, millet, oats, rice, rye, and wheat) and not-so-common grains (amaranth, farro, kamut, quinoa, sorghum, spelt, teff, and triticale). We highlight each grain's nourishing powers, and provide a four-week diet plan, with delicious menu ideas, and 50 recipes to teach you how to make wholegrains an integral part of your healthy lifestyle.

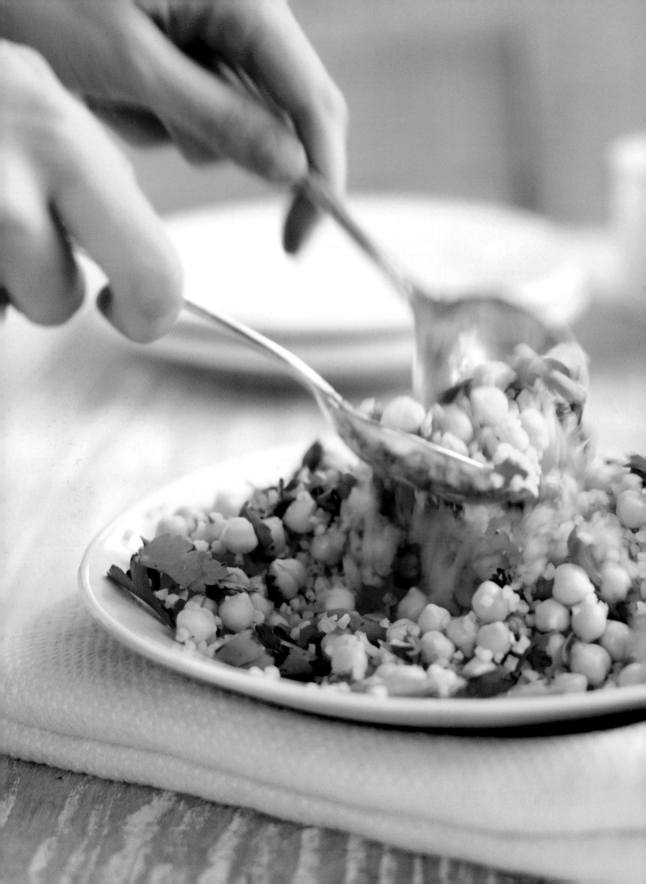

health benefits

why eat wholegrains?

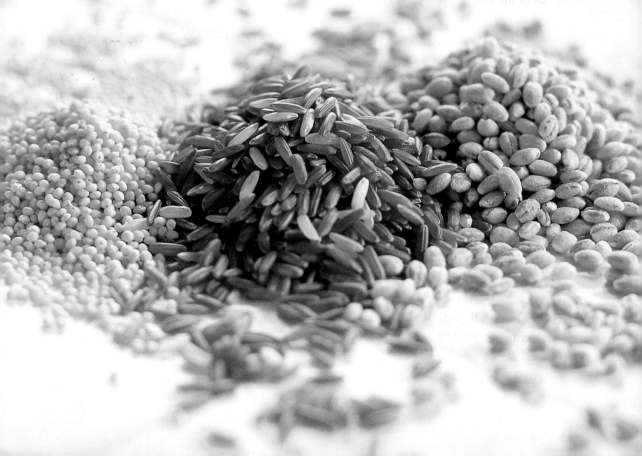

wholegrains for better health

1 Wholegrains in their natural state, unlike refined grains, are a rich source of fibre, vitamins, minerals, disease-protective antioxidants and phytochemicals. A large number of scientific studies have already identified significant health benefits from eating wholegrains, but the full benefits are still being discovered.

2 A wholegrain diet is effective and sustainable for long-term weight loss. Wholegrains are high in fibre and they have a low GI rating, which means they don't promote sudden spikes in blood sugar levels. This keeps insulin levels low, meaning less fat is stored and you are less hungry between meals.

3 Studies show that the high fibre content and protective antioxidant properties of wholegrains may reduce the risk of pancreatic, stomach, and colorectal cancer by 20–40 per cent, as well as reducing the risk of breast, uterine, and ovarian cancers.

4 Eating wholegrains may lower the risk of heart disease – the most common cause of death in the UK. Research shows that eating wholegrains daily can reduce blood pressure, lower "bad" cholesterol, and raise "good" cholesterol, which all contribute to reducing the risk of, and possibly preventing, heart disease.

5 Consuming wholegrains regularly can reduce the risk of developing type 2 diabetes. They can also be an important part of treatment for diabetics. The fibre in wholegrains may improve (or help to maintain) insulin sensitivity, thereby reducing the risk of developing glucose intolerance, or "pre-diabetes".

6 The fibre in wholegrains is beneficial for people who suffer from gastrointestinal problems. Eating more fibre-rich wholegrains can help to ease the discomfort associated with constipation and haemorrhoids. If you have coeliac disease, including gluten-free wholegrains in your diet can help prevent inflammatory reactions.

FACTS

Nine out of ten
adults in the UK fail to eat the recommended three servings of wholegrains per day.

•

One in three
adults in the UK do not even eat one portion of wholegrains each day.

•

People who eat
wholegrains tend to eat less and, consequently, weigh less too.

•

Just one serving
of wholegrains per day is enough to reduce blood pressure, lower "bad" cholesterol, and raise "good" cholesterol.

•

You can reduce the risk
of diseases such as type 2 diabetes and certain types of cancer by 20–40 per cent by eating wholegrains on a regular basis.

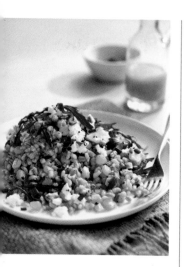

sweetcorn, barley, and rocket salad with goat's cheese (*see pp96–97*).

weight control

Despite the recent popularity of "low-carb" fad diets, nutrition experts have long said that for weight control not all carbs are "bad". In fact, over the past 10 years numerous studies have documented the link between wholegrain intake and a reduced risk of obesity. Research shows that countries with the highest fibre consumption have the lowest rates of obesity. Fibre and breakfast intake have also been linked to a lower body mass index level (BMI – the ratio of your weight to your height).

Fibre and reduced hunger

People who eat wholegrains regularly tend to eat less, which is probably why they also often weigh less. In an ongoing study (of women), researchers concluded that "women who consumed more wholegrains consistently weighed less than women who consumed less." Part of the explanation for this may lie in the fact that many wholegrains are excellent sources of fibre, and studies have shown that high fibre intake is associated with less hunger. Wholegrains are also higher in protein than refined grains and, as protein takes longer to digest than carbohydrates alone, this can result in a reduction of hunger.

Studies have also demonstrated that if you eat wholegrains for breakfast, you will eat less food at lunch and dinner. In fact, one study shows that a cereal and milk meal twice a day with a healthy lunch is as effective for weight loss as taking a meal replacement shake. According to the US National Weight Control Registry, an ongoing study of people who have lost weight and kept it off, 80 per cent of these successful dieters eat breakfast. So, if you're not a breakfast eater, it's time to start. If you are, consider breakfast as an ideal opportunity to add wholegrains to your diet.

Calories and low-fat diets

The "calorific density" of wholegrains is low. That means that you can eat more of them and feel less hungry, while at the same time, taking fewer calories in. Calorific density of a food is determined by its fat, fibre, and water content. Wholegrains are high in fibre and low in fat and therefore have a low calorific density.

Many studies have shown that lower calorific density diets are associated with reduced calorie intake. In a review of existing scientific studies, nutritionists have shown that more weight is lost on a diet that is high in fibre and low in fat than on a diet that is only low in fat. This may be because low-fat diets are not very "filling", and that adding fibre restores the diets' "satiety" (ability to make you feel full).

Insulin: the hunger hormone

Insulin, a hormone secreted by the pancreas, is responsible for transporting sugar out of the bloodstream and into the cells of the body. High insulin levels are also responsible for causing an increase in hunger (since blood sugar levels are low).

As insulin secretion is stimulated by eating sugar and carbohydrates, low-carbohydrate diets have become an extremely popular method for inducing a quick-fix weight loss. The idea is that if you avoid eating carbohydrates, you reduce your secretion of insulin and reduce hunger, while promoting weight loss. Whilst, in theory, correct, the long-term health effects of low-carbohydrate diets are unknown. What's more worrying is that they may even be harmful, particularly for the kidneys.

The weight you lose will be kept off because this diet works better the longer you follow it.

However, a low-GI (glycaemic index) diet, rich in wholegrains, may produce similar weight loss results, but without the health risks associated with most low carbohydrate diets. Because wholegrains are high in fibre, they have a lower GI rating, which means they yield a small effect on blood sugar levels. The fibre reduces the amount of sugar the body can absorb from a carbohydrate, leading to lower insulin levels. Lower levels of insulin mean that less fat is stored and you are also less hungry between meals.

Long-term weight control

Wholegrains represent a logical, healthy, and effective way to control your weight in the long term. In an ongoing study of men who were not actively trying to lose weight, the more wholegrains eaten by the participants, the more weight they lost over time. In fact, after eight years, their weight was about one kilogram (2lb) lower for every 40 grams (1½oz) of wholegrains eaten each day. In short, the weight that you lose on a wholegrain diet will be kept off because this diet works better the longer you follow it.

BOTTOM LINE

People who eat wholegrains tend to eat less, which may be why they often weigh less.

•

Research suggests that if you eat wholegrains at breakfast, you will eat less food at lunch and dinner.

•

Wholegrains are high in fibre and have a low GI rating, which means they don't promote spikes in blood sugar levels.

•

The "calorific density" of wholegrains is low, which means you can eat more of them, whilst also taking fewer calories in.

•

A wholegrain diet is an effective way to control weight as it works best in the long term.

•

Studies have shown that the more wholegrains you eat, the more weight you are likely to lose over time.

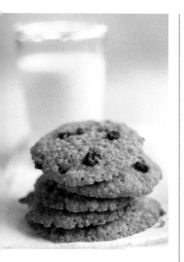

oatmeal raisin cookies
(*see pp150–51*).

heart disease

Heart disease is the most common cause of death (including premature death) in the UK. On average, one British adult dies from the disease every three minutes, accounting for approximately one in five deaths in men and one in six deaths in women each year. Just under 2.7 million people in the UK suffer from some form of heart disease and it is estimated to cost the UK nearly £8 billion a year in healthcare, informal care, and productivity losses.

Prevention is key

During the last 20 years, increased public awareness of the role of diet and exercise, improved screening and early detection of heart disease, and more aggressive treatment of risk factors, such as high blood pressure and high cholesterol, have led to a decline in the number of deaths from these diseases. However, the high number of people still dying from heart disease means prevention must remain a priority.

Reducing the risk of heart disease

Many factors are known to increase your risk of developing heart disease; some you cannot control, others you can. Your age, gender, family history, and genetic makeup cannot be altered, but you can reduce their impact with proper diet and exercise. By adopting a healthier lifestyle, which includes eating healthily every day, controlling your weight and blood pressure, being physically active, and avoiding or quitting cigarette smoking, you can reduce your risk and possibly prevent heart disease.

Major risk factors for heart disease:

- Elevated LDL ("bad") cholesterol levels
- Elevated total cholesterol levels
- Low HDL ("good") cholesterol levels
- Type 2 diabetes
- Cigarette smoking and exposure to tobacco smoke
- High blood pressure
- Family history of premature heart disease
- Age (men older than 45 years; women older than 55 years)
- Obesity (BMI greater than 30)
- Sedentary lifestyle (inadequate exercise)

Wholegrains and heart disease

One study on the relationship between dietary fibre intake and the risk of heart disease found that in men, the chance of having a heart attack differed depending on how much fibre they ate every day. For the group with the highest dietary fibre intake (about 30 grams/1oz per day) the risk was nearly half that of men in the lowest group, who ate only about 12 grams (just under ½oz) per day. Importantly, cereal fibre was found to be most strongly associated with a reduced risk of a heart attack.

Researchers have found that a diet containing oats and buckwheat is linked to a lowered risk of high blood pressure and high cholesterol, respectively. Only one 85 gram (3oz) serving per day of each grain was needed to reduce blood pressure, lower total and LDL ("bad") cholesterol, and raise HDL ("good") cholesterol. Another study reviewing the diets of women between the ages of 55 and 69 years found that the higher a woman's intake of wholegrains, the lower her risk of heart disease. Conversely, the higher the intake of refined grains, the higher the risk of heart disease.

Studies show the more wholegrains people eat, the lower their risk of heart disease.

A study examining how much wholegrain, bran, and germ would reduce the risk of heart disease found that the more wholegrains participants ate, the lower their risk of heart disease. The reverse was also true: those who ate the least amount of wholegrains had the highest risk. The association was even stronger for bran, possibly suggesting that bran may contain the most biologically active components in the fight against heart disease.

Dietary advice

Taken together, these studies, along with many others, clearly establish the benefits of wholegrains in reducing the risk of heart disease. But it is important to keep in mind that dietary saturated fat and cholesterol also need to be limited to reduce your risk of heart disease. Major sources of saturated fat and cholesterol in the diet include fatty meats, butter, cheese, cream, and whole milk. Replace saturated fats with foods rich in monounsaturated fats (olive oil, nuts, avocado), polyunsaturated fats (fish, vegetables oils, seeds), and plant foods (beans, legumes, wholegrains).

BOTTOM LINE

By adopting a healthier lifestyle – eating healthily, controlling your weight and blood pressure, and exercising regularly – you can reduce your risk of, and possibly prevent, heart disease.

●

Replace saturated fat with monounsaturated fats (found in olive oil and nuts) and polyunsaturated fats (found in fish and vegetable oils).

●

Numerous studies show that the higher the intake of wholegrains, the lower the risk of heart disease.

●

Conversely, studies show that the lower the intake of wholegrains (and the higher the intake of refined grains), the higher the risk of heart disease.

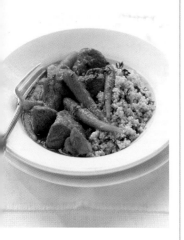

veal stew with millet, baby carrots, and thyme (*see pp128–29*).

cancer

Cancer is a group of diseases characterized by the uncontrolled growth and spread of abnormal cells. Although mortality rates are decreasing, cancer is among the three leading causes of death at all ages except pre-school children in the UK. There are many different types of cancers, and the disease can affect organs (such as the colon or prostate) as well as tissues (such as blood or bone). The most common types of cancer in the UK are breast, skin, lung, colorectal (large bowel), and prostate.

The role of environmental factors

Researchers have been working hard to uncover the links between diet and various forms of cancer. Unfortunately, because cancer is the result of an extremely complicated process that develops over time, scientists have not been able to clearly determine its exact causes. Early studies have, however, identified links between environmental factors, such as high levels of fat in the diets of certain populations and cancer risk.

In the UK, it is believed that up to 12,000 people yearly could avoid developing cancer by maintaining a healthy lifestyle. Research also suggests that about a third of cancer deaths in the US each year are associated with poor nutrition, physical inactivity, and obesity. Studies indicate that obese people have a higher risk of developing cancer and dying from it. The types of cancers more frequently linked with excess weight in women are breast, uterine, cervical, and ovarian, and for men, prostate, stomach, and colorectal.

A complicated relationship

Wholegrains may help to reduce the risk of some cancers, but the reasons for this are not clear cut. One problem with the information these studies provide is that much of the research focuses on dietary fibre (rather than wholegrains specifically), which can be found in a range of foods, including wholegrains, but also fruits and vegetables. All of these high-fibre foods are part of a healthy diet, so trying to determine which group (or which component) has what effect on the development of cancer, has been difficult to isolate. In addition, the relationship of fibre and cancers in different tissues is complex and still being researched. In short, the regular inclusion of wholegrains in the diet appears to help prevent the development of cancers, but researchers are not yet sure why.

Fibre and cancer

Research suggests that dietary fibre may help to reduce the risk of gastrointestinal cancers (such as colon, stomach, etc.). One possible explanation for this is that the fibre (in wholegrains, for example) increases faecal bulk and this reduces transit time (makes you go to the bathroom sooner) and thus is expected to reduce the exposure of intestinal cells to potential cancer-causing chemicals found in our diet.

Numerous studies have confirmed a link between the intake of wholegrains and the risk of specific types of cancer. For example, two independent studies both concluded that increased fibre intake could lower the risk of colon or rectum cancer, pancreatic cancer, and stomach cancer by 20–40 per cent.

Phytochemicals and cancer

Studies in the US have shown that cancers of the uterus and ovaries are less likely to occur in women who eat wholegrains on a daily basis. One US study documented almost 40 per cent fewer uterine cancers in women who ate one to two servings of wholegrains per day, compared to those who didn't. Some researchers believe that this protective effect is, in fact, due to the phytoestrogens (a plant-derived cousin of the human sex hormone) that wholegrains contain, and not necessarily a product of its fibre.

Phytoestrogens are believed to protect hormone-sensitive tissues (such as the breast and uterus) by binding to the oestrogen receptors and blocking the binding of natural oestrogen. According to this theory, too much natural oestrogen is part of the root cause of certain types of cancer. Experiments continue in an effort to discover exactly how wholegrains exert their protective effects and how powerful these effects are.

Continued research

It remains to be determined whether it is the fibre in wholegrains that is protective, or if it is the phytochemicals and antioxidants that protect the cells in the body.

It is important to determine these mechanisms because each grain has different components that will determine the specific health benefits. For instance, in a study published by S. van Rensburg in 1981 comparing rates of cancer from different parts of the world, researchers found that in places where sorghum or millet was eaten, oesophageal cancer rates were lower than in places where wheat or corn were more popular. They provided convincing evidence that the risk of oesophageal cancer was related to nutrient deficiencies that were prevented in those consuming millet or sorghum.

BOTTOM LINE

As many as 12,000 people a year in the UK could avoid developing cancer by adopting and maintaining a healthy lifestyle.

•

Studies have shown that people who are obese have a higher risk of developing cancer.

•

Eating wholegrains could lower the risk of colorectal, pancreatic, and stomach cancers by 20–40 per cent.

•

Cancers of the uterus and ovaries are less likely to occur in women who eat wholegrains on a daily basis.

•

Research suggests that the nutrients provided by sorghum or millet may help to protect against oesophageal cancer.

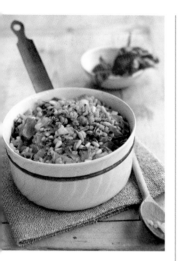

barley with leeks and
fennel (*see pp132–33*).

type 2 diabetes

Diabetes is defined by an abnormally high level of sugar, or glucose, in the blood. The most common types of diabetes are type 1 and type 2. Type 1 develops suddenly and results from an allergy-like response in the body. Type 1 diabetics don't have the ability to produce insulin. Type 2 diabetes is affected by diet and obesity, and it develops over time. Sadly, type 2 diabetes is becoming a global epidemic, but incorporating wholegrains into your diet can help prevent the condition.

Who is at risk?

Type 1 diabetes usually starts in childhood and used to be called Juvenile Diabetes. Type 2 diabetes, on the other hand, is associated with an over-production of insulin, which is due to a decreased response to insulin's action in the body. Type 2 diabetes is much more common and is more likely to develop in those who are overweight or obese. While Type 2 diabetes was once referred to as Adult-Onset Diabetes, it has now been reported in children under the age of 10 years old.

Pre-conditions for type 2 diabetes

Type 2 diabetes does not develop overnight. Before people develop the condition, they almost always have "pre-diabetes" or "glucose intolerance", where the body's ability to respond to carbohydrate (especially simple sugars) is impaired and "insulin resistance" develops (abnormal insulin secretion). Eventually these abnormalities lead to type 2 diabetes. Wholegrains can influence both glucose intolerance and insulin resistance and can therefore be an important part of treatment for diabetics, as well as a means of prevention.

Fibre and blood sugar control

The link between the fibre contained in wholegrains and blood sugar control is not a new concept. Denis Burkitt and Hugh Trowell's "fibre hypothesis" documented the beneficial relationship between type 2 diabetes and fibre intake in the 1970s. James Anderson (another early proponent of the fibre hypothesis) published an article in 1979, describing how fibre exerts its important effects in the body. Since these publications, literally hundreds of scientific studies have examined the fibre hypothesis and confirmed many of the theorized benefits of fibre. The exact mechanism by which fibre affects the body is still under active investigation, but in general, these studies show a 20–40 per cent reduced risk of diabetes in those who regularly eat wholegrains. Results from one study showed that people who ate the most wholegrains had the lowest insulin levels and the greatest insulin sensitivity. Other studies show that the larger the particle size of the grain, the longer it takes to digest and the slower the rise in blood glucose levels after the grain is eaten. This leads to lower insulin levels and improves (or helps to maintain) insulin sensitivity.

Those grains high in soluble fibre, such as oats, rye, and barley, have been shown to be more effective at improving insulin sensitivity than grains high in insoluble fibre, such as wholewheat and buckwheat. Other grains, such as corn and rice with minimal fibre content, did not have much of an impact on insulin sensitivity. This has led some investigators to compare the effects of various grains that contain different amounts and types of fibre.

Wholegrains can influence both glucose intolerance and insulin resistance.

Replacing insoluble fibre with more soluble fibre can significantly decrease both blood sugar and cholesterol levels. For example, one study looking at different types of fibre, replaced a group of type 2 diabetics' typical corn and rice-based cereals with wheat and oat-based cereals with added psyllium (for an even greater soluble-fibre boost). Over the next three months, participants exhibited reduced blood triglyceride levels (a type of fat in the blood that increases after you eat food) and improvements in the ratio of total to HDL ("good") cholesterol levels. The study's conclusion was that, over time, as these diabetic subjects adapted to a higher fibre intake, their risk of heart disease decreased.

A combined effect

In addition to being high in fibre, wholegrains are also an excellent source of magnesium, and many researchers believe that this mineral may too play a role in the prevention and treatment of type 2 diabetes. So, currently, it is unclear whether it is the fibre or the magnesium in wholegrains that confer the benefits related to type 2 diabetes. The most likely conclusion is that it is probably a combination of the two. We can just be happy that wholegrains work, without worrying about how.

BOTTOM LINE

The risk of type 2 diabetes is 20–40 per cent lower in those with a higher wholegrain intake, compared to those who eat very few wholegrains.

•

Higher fibre intake helps to control blood sugar levels in type 2 diabetics, which may reduce the quantity of medication needed.

•

Substituting high-fibre wholegrains for refined grains can improve insulin sensitivity, which may reduce the risk of developing type 2 diabetes.

•

Wholegrains are also rich in magnesium, and scientists believe that this mineral may play an important part in preventing and treating type 2 diabetes.

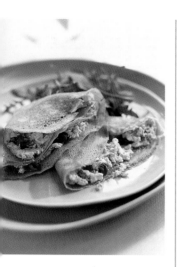

buckwheat crêpes with
goat's cheese and sun-
dried tomatoes (*see p110*).

metabolic syndrome

*Metabolic syndrome (or syndrome X) is a cluster of abnormalities
that combine to increase the risk of type 2 diabetes and heart disease.
The components include elevated blood pressure; increased waist
circumference – more than 100cm (40 inches) for a man or 87.5cm (35
inches) for a woman; glucose intolerance (also called "pre-diabetes");
elevated triglyceride levels (the most common form of fat present in
the blood) and low HDL ("good") cholesterol levels in the blood.*

Factors for metabolic syndrome

Metabolic syndrome may affect one in four people in the UK and the US.
The older you get, the more likely you are to develop metabolic syndrome,
so almost half of people over 60 years of age meet the criteria. Seventy-
five per cent of those with metabolic syndrome are overweight.

Many people with metabolic syndrome exhibit four key characteristics:
insulin resistance, excess abdominal weight, high blood pressure, and
abnormal blood lipid levels. (Other symptoms may include a fatty liver
and, in women, polycistic ovarian syndrome.) Each of the health
abnormalities, outlined below, on their own may not indicate a major
health problem, but when they occur concurrently, they are an indication
of risk of heart disease and type 2 diabetes. If you have any of these risk
factors, ask your doctor to screen you for metabolic syndrome.

Characteristics associated with metabolic syndrome:

- Insulin resistance
- Abdominal obesity
- Elevated blood pressure
- Abnormal blood lipid levels

Insulin resistance

A major component of metabolic syndrome is insulin resistance. Insulin,
a hormone produced by the pancreas, has a number of important roles in
the body, the most obvious of which is to help transport sugar from the
blood into the cells. Insulin resistance occurs when the body needs more
insulin than normal to do its job. In other words, when you eat carbohydrates,
your blood sugar level shoots up higher and stays high longer than is
considered normal.

Research shows that foods high in fibre, added to a low saturated fat diet, improve insulin sensitivity (thus reversing glucose intolerance). Therefore, the healthiest and most sustainable way to control insulin secretion (and to deal with insulin resistance) is by eating wholegrains and avoiding refined carbohydrates (such as white bread, cakes, and anything else made with refined flour or sugar).

This is considered to be a low-glycaemic (low-GI) way to eat. Unlike the low carbohydrate diets, which omit carbohydrates altogether, eating carbohydrates in the form of wholegrains has repeatedly been shown to be associated with better health outcomes. This is because wholegrains are digested more slowly, releasing their sugar into the blood stream in a steady, controlled fashion that allows the body to assimilate the sugar without secreting large amounts of insulin. One study has shown that cereal fibre from wholegrains was associated with protection against metabolic syndrome and that insulin sensitivity was exacerbated by an increased intake of refined carbohydrates.

Abdominal obesity

Excess abdominal fat, or fat stored around the belly, is the most significant factor contributing to insulin resistance and heart disease, and it is a key component in metabolic syndrome. Fortunately, with simple dietary and lifestyle changes, it is not very difficult to shed belly fat. Incorporating wholegrains into your diet, eating reasonable portion sizes, and exercising regularly, will promote the loss of abdominal fat, as this type of fat is usually the first fat lost when you embark on a weight loss regime.

Elevated blood pressure

High blood pressure (also known as hypertension) is another defining characteristic of metabolic syndrome, and it can contribute to heart disease, especially when combined with abdominal obesity. If you have high blood pressure, you should eat a low-fat diet, with wholegrains and lots of fruits and vegetables. Studies suggest that adding just two servings a day of soluble-fibre rich grains to your diet can help lower blood pressure.

Abnormal lipid levels

High lipid levels – specifically, high triglyceride levels (the most common form of fat in the blood) and low HDL ("good") cholesterol levels in the blood – are also associated with metabolic syndrome. Abnormal lipid levels may result from eating too many refined carbohydrates and too much sugar. To avoid high lipid levels, increase your intake of wholegrains and fibre-rich vegetables, exercise regularly, and avoid or quit smoking.

BOTTOM LINE

Metabolic syndrome is associated with high blood pressure, abdominal obesity, glucose intolerance, and abnormal lipid levels.

•

These health problems do not indicate a major problem on their own. However, if they occur concurrently, they may increase the risk of heart disease and diabetes.

•

Wholegrains are thought to improve insulin sensitivity (reversing glucose intolerance) and protect against type 2 diabetes.

•

Eating wholegrains as part of a low-fat diet and healthy lifestyle lowers blood pressure and helps to shed abdominal obesity, thereby reducing the risk of developing heart disease.

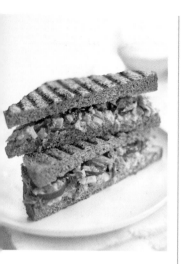

quinoa tuna salad
sandwich on wholemeal
bread (*see p111*).

gastrointestinal diseases

The gastrointestinal, or digestive, system is comprised of the gastronintestinal (GI) tract (a tube that runs from the mouth to the anus that is responsible for assimilating nutrients and eliminating bodily waste products) and its associated organs, such as the pancreas, liver, and gall bladder. These organs are important to nutrition because they are where nutrients are broken down and processed to be transported throughout the body for energy, growth, and repair.

The role of fibre in the GI tract

Scientists have determined that fibre plays a vital role in the health of the GI tract. There are two types of fibre: soluble and insoluble fibre. Soluble fibre (found in grains such as oats and barley) binds to water in the GI tract and creates a gel-like mixture. This gel slows the rate at which food leaves the stomach and glucose enters the bloodstream. It also blocks the absorption of bile acids, which helps to lower cholesterol levels.

Insoluble fibre (found in grains such as wholewheat and brown rice) create bulk in the intestinal tract, helping food to move through the gut more quickly. This reduces the calories available to be absorbed and causes a change in the type of bacteria present in the colon. These healthier bacteria reduce cancer-promoting compounds, which may explain the reduced risk of colon cancer associated with a high-fibre diet (*see Cancer, pp18–19*). Insoluble fibre can promote gas production, though, which may temporarily make you feel uncomfortable.

Easing constipation and haemorrhoids

Constipation is defined as the infrequent (fewer than three times per week) and difficult passage of stools that are small and hard, which may result in straining to have bowel movements. As many as 14 million people in the UK suffer from constipation, and it is usually due to a diet lacking in fibre. Fibre in food traps water and adds bulk to the stool, making it easier to move through the colon. A high-fibre diet – which includes wholegrains, vegetables, and fruits, in conjunction with exercise, and plenty of fluids – is usually very effective at relieving the symptoms of constipation.

While not a serious medical condition, haemorrhoids are very common and cause a great deal of worry and annoyance to those who have them. Although there is no strong evidence to suggest that haemorrhoids can be prevented with a high-fibre diet, it is certain that if you do have haemorrhoids, the presence of fibre in your diet will make your stool softer and easier to pass, thus making your haemorrhoids less likely to become inflamed and bleed.

Preventing diverticular diseases

Diverticulosis is the presence of small pouches (known as diverticuli) in the wall of the colon. These are commonly caused by constipation due to lack of fibre in the diet. Diverticulosis is common in countries such as the UK and US where the intake of fibre tends to be low, and as people age, it becomes increasingly common. In instances where symptoms are present, they may include mild abdominal cramps, bloating, or intermittent diarrhoea or constipation.

Often there are no symptoms, however, which means diverticulosis can go undetected and may develop into diverticulitis, a more serious condition. Diverticulitis is a condition when the diverticuli become inflamed and this can cause tenderness in the lower abdomen, fever, nausea, vomiting, chills, cramping, and constipation. The insoluble fibre in wholegrains helps keep stools soft and easy to pass and prevents constipation, reducing the risk of diverticulosis and diverticulitis.

Irritable Bowel Syndrome and fibre

Symptoms associated with Irritable Bowel Syndrome (IBS) are abdominal pain and bloating, with periods of constipation or diarrhoea. The causes of IBS are not clear, but some believe it may be linked to an overactivity in certain areas of the gut. IBS is the ultimate diagnosis of up to 50 per cent of patients referred to gastroenterologists and, in the UK, up to one in five people will develop IBS at some point in their life. The fibre in wholegrains prevents constipation, and can thereby benefit those with IBS.

Reducing the risk of gallstones

Gallstones are formed from bile, a cholesterol-rich liquid made by the liver and stored in the gall bladder that aids the digestive process. When the bile in the gall bladder has an excess concentration of cholesterol and becomes thickened into sludge, small and then larger stones can eventually form. Gallstones are more common in people over 40, and in those who are overweight or eat a high-fat diet.

Populations that eat less fat and more fibre tend to have lower risks of gallstones, as do those who weigh less. Thus wholegrains may play a role both in preventing gallstones by helping with weight control and also by binding bile acids and leading to cholesterol excretion.

BOTTOM LINE

There are two types of dietary fibre, soluble and insoluble.

•

The fibre in wholegrains can help to ease the discomfort associated with gastrointestinal diseases.

•

As many as 14 million people in the UK suffer from constipation.

•

A high-fibre diet, which includes wholegrains, can be very effective at relieving the symptoms of constipation.

•

Fibre from wholegrains will make faeces softer and easier to pass, meaning haemorrhoids are less likely to become inflamed and bleed.

•

Wholegrains may help to prevent gallstones by assisting in cholesterol excretion and weight loss.

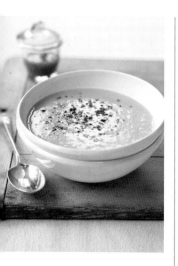

hearty millet and butternut
squash soup
(*see pp92–93*).

coeliac disease

Wholegrains are especially healthful foods, but there are some people who cannot tolerate certain grains. Coeliac disease (also called non-tropical sprue, or gluten intolerance) is an autoimmune disease, where the body produces antibodies that attack its own tissues. For people with coeliac disease, this attack is triggered by gluten (a protein found in some grains). It causes damage to the small intestine, which becomes inflamed and inhibits the proper absorption of food.

What is coeliac disease?

Coeliac disease is a genetic disease, which runs in families and occurs in both children and adults. It is estimated that 125,000 people have been diagnosed with coeliac disease in the UK. However, recent studies show that 1 in 100 people suffer from coeliac disease, which means there are almost another 500,000 people who remain undiagnosed. Wheat, rye, and barley are the most common offenders, with oats being a bit controversial. This is because, although oats do not contain gluten, they can trigger reactions in those with a gluten sensitivity (possibly because oats often become contaminated with wheat flour before they are purchased).

The classic symptoms

Exposure to gluten protein causes an inflammatory reaction in the cells lining the intestines of sensitive individuals. This leads to reduced absorption of calories and nutrients from food and may be experienced as abdominal pain, gas, bloating, cramping, and diarrhoea.

Coeliac disease usually develops early in life (most often in infants and in children younger than five years old), but it can occur at any age. In infants, the classic signs of coeliac disease may surface within months of the introduction of wheat into a baby's diet and, if left untreated, it can cause growth failure.

Other people may develop coeliac disease later in life as adults or young adults. For example, coeliac disease has been diagnosed in girls who are late getting their first period or whose menstrual cycles are irregular. When individuals develop gluten sensitivity at a later stage in life, they are likely to begin to experience abdominal complaints including, but not limited to, recurrent abdominal pain, nausea, vomiting, bloating, and constipation.

Silent coeliac disease

While coeliac disease was initially believed to be restricted to those who had severe digestive problems and weight loss, more recently "silent" forms of coeliac disease have been recognized. People with "silent" coeliac disease may have no symptoms at all for many years. Some complaints entail no intestinal symptoms, but lethargy or anaemia, while others may resemble the symptoms of irritable bowel syndrome (alternating constipation and diarrhoea). However, if coeliac disease is left undiagnosed (and therefore untreated), it can progress and eventually symptoms may appear due to nutritional deficiency.

Getting tested

If you suspect that you have a problem digesting certain grains, or if you have symptoms that your doctor cannot explain, ask your doctor for an anti-gliadin antibody blood test. Since this is a genetic problem, family members of those who have been diagnosed should also be tested, even if there are no symptoms present. Gluten-free diets may improve the symptoms, heal existing damage, and prevent further intestinal deterioration. Improvement begins within days of starting the diet, and the small intestine is usually healed and working properly in three to six months. For older adults, recovery may take up to two years. This gluten-free diet should be continued for life.

Although coeliac disease may be difficult to recognize – because we may not think immediately about coeliac disease when experiencing some of these symptoms, or the disease may be silent – the problems are reversible with the adoption of a gluten-free diet. The good news is that there are still many delicious wholegrains that can be eaten even by those on a gluten-free diet, as shown below. Each grain profile in this book tells you whether or not it is safe for those with coeliac disease and the resources section (*see pp156–57*) includes information on locating and buying gluten-free wholegrain products.

Grains to enjoy:
- Amaranth
- Buckwheat
- Corn
- Millet
- Quinoa
- Rice
- Sorghum
- Teff

Grains to avoid:
- Barley
- Farro
- Kamut
- Oats
- Rye
- Spelt
- Triticale
- Wheat (including bulgur)

BOTTOM LINE

Studies show that 1 in 100 people in the UK suffer from coeliac disease (also known as gluten intolerance).

•

For people with coeliac disease, gluten causes the intestine to become inflamed leading to a reduced absorption of calories and nutrients from food.

•

A gluten-free diet (including wholegrains such as amaranth, quinoa, and buckwheat) may improve the symptoms of coeliac disease and prevent further damage.

•

Because coeliac disease is genetic, family members of those who have been diagnosed should be tested even if they have no symptoms.

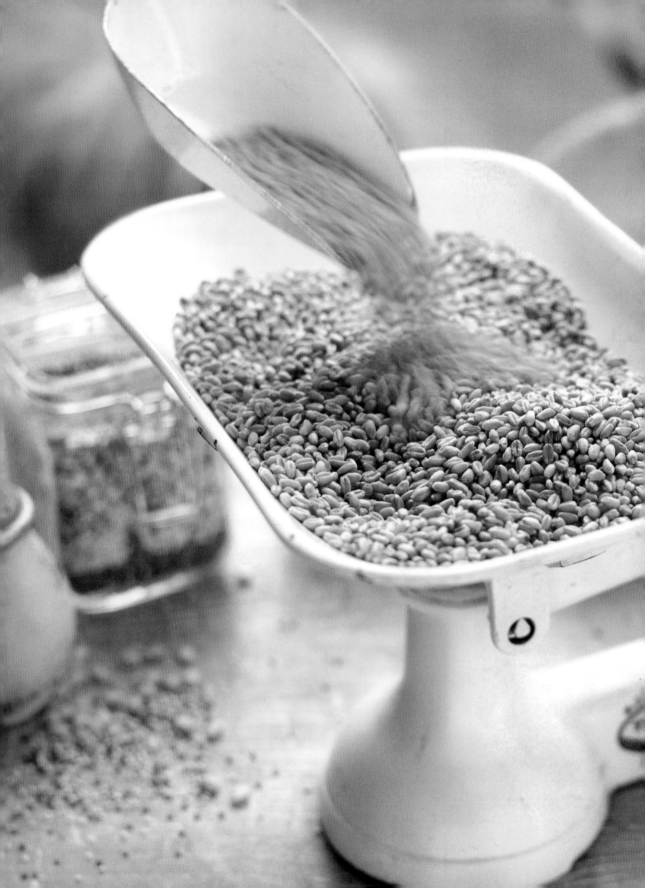

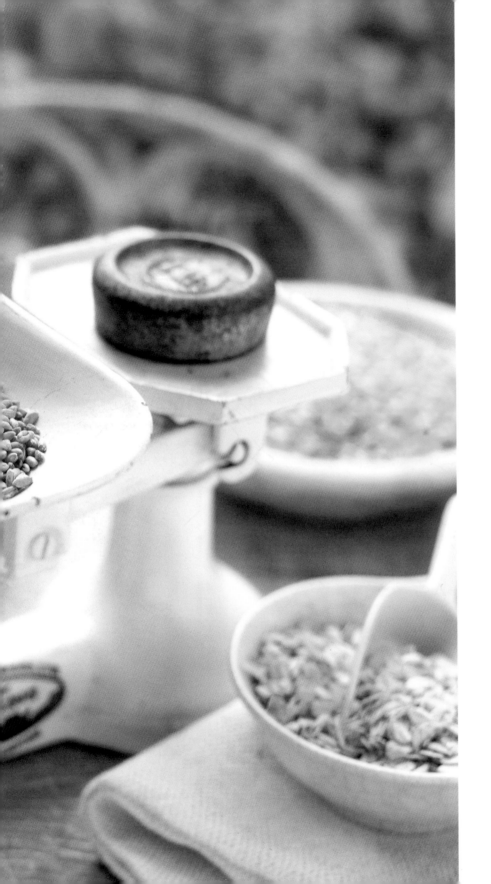

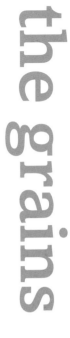
the grains

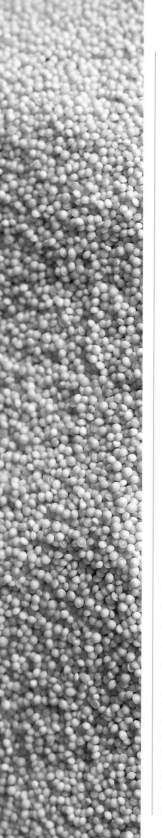

amaranth

Once revered by the Aztecs, amaranth became a "lost" seed for many generations. Interest in amaranth was revived in the 1970s, due to the recognition of its superior nutritional qualities, hardiness, and great taste. It is now cultivated commercially throughout South America, South Asia, and the United States, and is enjoyed worldwide.

History

Amaranth is a seed with a gory past: the ancient Aztecs believed that amaranth seeds bore supernatural powers and represented human sacrifice. Aztec women mixed amaranth seeds with honey and human blood to shape idols that were eaten as part of religious ceremonies. When the Conquistadors confronted the Aztec civilization in the early 16th century, they were horrified by the practice of consuming blood and sacrificing humans. Believing they could stop these practices by outlawing amaranth, the Spanish prohibited the cultivation of the seed, and it fell into obscurity. (This political decision is believed to have contributed to the ultimate demise of the Aztec culture.) Fortunately, the grain thrived in a few remote areas of the Andes and Mexico without human cultivation, and grew wild for centuries.

Centuries later amaranth experienced a renaissance in South America, and it is now an integral part of many cultures' ceremonies and daily diets. In Mexico, amaranth seeds are popped and served as a sweetened dessert. In Peru, women adorn themselves with amaranth flowers and bundles during their annual carnival. Amaranth seeds are eaten and the flowers are celebrated for their striking beauty in other countries throughout the world. Since 1975, amaranth has been gaining popularity in the United States, and although it is not yet a mainstream food, it is becoming more widely available to people worldwide.

Description

Not a true grain, amaranth is actually a hardy, bushy, flowering plant that can grow as tall as two metres (about seven feet) and is able to withstand both drought and extreme heat. The flowers of the amaranth plant are red or magenta in colour and contain thousands of tiny edible seeds. The seeds can be boiled and eaten as a cereal, milled into flour, sprouted, toasted, or popped like popcorn. Boiled amaranth has a sticky texture that contrasts with the fluffier texture of many grains and its flavour is nutty and slightly sweet. The nutrients in amaranth seeds are concentrated in a natural "ring" that surrounds the central starchy section, protecting the nutrients during harvesting and processing.

Cooking amaranth

To prepare amaranth seeds, use three parts water to one part amaranth. Add the amaranth to boiling water (approximately 15–20 minutes), until the water is absorbed. The seeds will feel tender and slightly sticky.

You can use amaranth flour to make a variety of baked goods and pastas. Because it is gluten-free, amaranth flour must be mixed with flours that are rich in gluten, such as wholewheat flour, when baking yeast breads. This is because gluten gives dough its elasticity, and, when baking, this elasticity allows the bread to rise without crumbling. However, in the preparation of pastas, flatbreads, or pancakes, 100 per cent amaranth flour can be used on its own.

One of the easiest ways to incorporate amaranth into your diet is to add the seed to soups or stews as a healthy thickening agent. Sprouting amaranth seeds will increase the level of some of the nutrients, and they can be added to dishes, or eaten as they are. Rinse the seeds thoroughly, and soak for 2–4 hours. Drain the seeds, put them in a jar covered with muslin, and place the jar in a sunny location, such as a windowsill. Rinse and drain the seeds every 12 hours; they should sprout in 24–48 hours.

Nutritional content

Amaranth seeds contain carbohydrates, protein, B vitamins, folate, phosphorus, calcium, magnesium, and potassium. Amaranth also has a higher level of protein than most other grains, and is particularly high in the amino acid, lysine (often in short supply in grains). Weight for weight, amaranth contains more calcium than milk and provides almost twice as much iron as wheat. Amaranth is an excellent source of fibre as well.

Health benefits

Amaranth is a good source of tocotrienols (a form of vitamin E), which have been shown to lower blood cholesterol levels. Additionally, amaranth contains heart-healthy polyunsaturated oil, which is found mostly within the germ, or inner layer, of the seed. This oil is high in linoleic acid (an essential fatty acid), which is thought to promote the body's anti-inflammatory process and prevent blood clotting. Amaranth has the added benefit of being gluten-free, and is therefore appropriate for anyone with coeliac disease or gluten intolerance.

FACTS

Strengthen your bones with amaranth, as it contains more calcium than milk.

•

The heart-healthy oils amaranth contains may help to lower blood cholesterol levels.

•

Amaranth provides nearly twice as much iron as wheat, and also contains more protein than most grains.

•

A gluten-free seed, amaranth is suitable for those who have coeliac disease or are gluten intolerant.

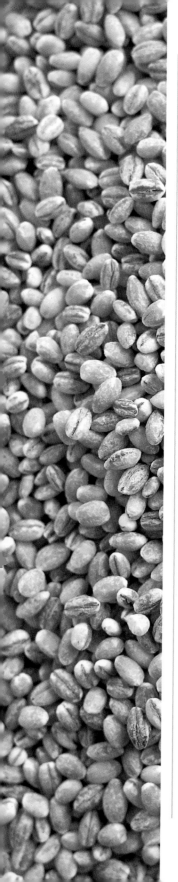

barley

One of the oldest grains in history, barley has served many purposes for different cultures – as a food for humans and animals, a staple to make beer, and even as currency in Babylonian times. Available year-round, the largest global producers of barley are Canada, the United States, Russia, Germany, France, and Spain.

History

Originally from Ethiopia and Southeast Asia, barley has been used in recipes dating as far back as 2800 BC. Even the Bible refers to barley in breads made by the Hebrews, Romans, and Greeks. In addition, the Chinese have been cooking with barley for more than 4,000 years. During the 16th century, barley was brought to South America by the Spanish and to the United States by English and Dutch settlers. Most likely, barley made its way to North America because of its ability to germinate and produce malt, a key ingredient for the production of beer.

Description

Barley is available in a number of forms, including hulled, pearled, hull-less, and flaked (*see below*). The grain consists of two outer husks, called the spikelet, which surround the cells of the endosperm. When barley is milled, the outer husks are removed, leaving the endosperm and making the grain edible. All variations require some processing, and even the most processed variety, heavily pearled barley, retains 50 per cent of its original fibre content after the bran is removed.

Hulled barley has only its outer coating removed, and has the highest nutritional content of any barley product. The bran, which remains untouched, contains the majority of barley's fibre, vitamins, and minerals.

Lightly pearled barley is not technically a wholegrain (as small amounts of the bran are missing), however it is full of fibre and much healthier than a fully refined grain. Choose this light-brown barley over the highly processed heavily pearled barley, which resembles white rice. Heavily pearled barley is, however, still rich in fibre (as unlike other grains, barley contains fibre throughout its kernel) but it is lacking in some of the other important nutrients that the less processed varieties contain.

Hull-less barley produces a hull that is loosely adhered to the kernel. This loose outer coating falls off of the kernel during harvesting, so minimal pearling is required.

Cracked barley or barley flakes are flattened and sliced barley kernels, typically made from hulled barley which has the bran intact. They look similar to rolled oats and may be used for cereals.

Barley flour is usually made from grinding barley, and can be blended with wholewheat flour when baking. Look for flour made from hulled or hull-less rather than pearled barley. Although it is not gluten-free, barley does have a relatively low gluten content, so barley flour may be a good choice for those wishing to minimize the amount of gluten in their diet.

Cooking barley
With its sweet, nutty flavour, barley is a tasty addition to everything from soups to salads, breads to cereals. When preparing any type of barley, add one part barley to three and a half parts boiling water. Once the liquid is boiling, reduce heat, cover, and simmer for about 45–60 minutes for pearled barley or 90 minutes for hulled barley.

Nutritional content
Barley contains carbohydrates and protein, soluble and insoluble fibre, and is a rich source of thiamin, niacin, selenium, iron, zinc, phosphorus, copper, and manganese. One serving of cooked barley contains about 50 per cent of the daily requirements for selenium, an important trace mineral required for normal thyroid hormone metabolism, antioxidant defence systems, and immune function. Selenium has also been shown to reduce the risk of developing cancer. All barley is rich in fibre and although pearled barley is processed, it still contains a significant amount of fibre. Barley is not suitable in the diets of people who are allergic to gluten.

Health benefits
The majority of the studies looking at the health benefits of barley have been conducted in conjunction with other wholegrains. Barley contains insoluble fibre, which cannot be digested, but has a bulking effect on stools that keeps the intestines in good condition. It also provides soluble fibre, which helps to regulate the absorption of glucose into the bloodstream. Barley's benefits are likely to be due to its high soluble and insoluble fibre content, as well as to the antioxidant properties of selenium. Thus, eating barley may help to prevent both heart disease and cancer.

FACTS

High in fibre, barley may help to reduce the risk of heart disease and cancer.

One serving of barley supplies half the daily requirement for selenium, which is thought to strengthen the immune system.

Hulled barley is the least processed and most nutritious variety of barley, as only its outer coating is removed.

Heavily pearled barley is more highly processed than other varieties, but it is still high in fibre, which is contained throughout the grain's kernel.

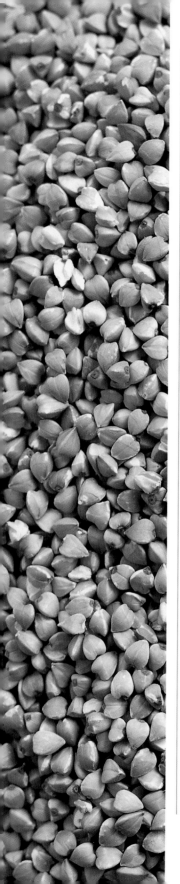

buckwheat

Despite its name, buckwheat is not actually related to wheat at all. This flowering plant, once used only as animal feed and fertilizer, has now become a staple for bakers, beekeepers, and health-conscious cooks. Soba noodles, made from buckwheat, are popular in Japanese cooking and also as an alternative to traditional pasta.

History

Originally cultivated in Central Asia and China in the 10th century, buckwheat made its way to Europe via migrations of people from Siberia and Manchuria. Because of its versatility, buckwheat became a mainstay in the cuisines of Finland, Austria, northern Italy, France, Russia, and Eastern Europe. German and Dutch settlers brought buckwheat to the United States in the 17th century and planted expansive fields throughout the state of New York. Beekeepers soon noticed that the fragrant nectar of the buckwheat blossom allowed bees to produce honey with an intense, delectable flavour.

Description

Buckwheat is a herbaceous plant from the Polygonaceae family. Unlike most other grains, it does not grow as a grass, but as a low-lying, flowering plant. Buckwheat is not a true grain, but it is actually a seed that is closely related to sorrel and rhubarb.

Raw groats are light brown in colour and have a mild, slightly bitter flavour. Raw groats are buckwheat kernels that are stripped of their outer, inedible hull and compressed into small pieces. To remove their bitter flavour, raw groats may be roasted in oil for several minutes until they achieve a deep, rust colour.

Roasted groats, also known as kasha, are dark brown in colour, with an intense, nutty flavour and aroma. They are usually toasted in oil and can be used to make pilaf, bread, and hot cereal.

Buckwheat cereal is made from ground buckwheat groats. It cooks quickly when boiled and is eaten as a hot cereal. Other names for buckwheat cereal are cream of buckwheat and buckwheat grits.

Buckwheat flour can be used to make noodles, pancakes, breads, muffins, crackers, tortillas, and biscuits. Available in both light and dark varieties, opt for the darker buckwheat flour whenever possible, as it is more nutritious. Buckwheat flour can be mixed with wholewheat flour to give baked products a distinctive, nutty flavour. (When substituting buckwheat flour for flours that contain gluten, such as plain or wholewheat, reduce the flour measurements by one half to two-thirds.)

Cooking buckwheat

Before cooking, rinse buckwheat briefly under cool, running water to remove any debris. If you are using raw groats, toast them lightly in oil until they reach a deep brown colour. To cook, add one part buckwheat to two parts boiling water or reduced-sodium broth. Once the liquid returns to a boil, turn down the heat, cover, and simmer for 15–20 minutes.

Buckwheat is a very porous seed and has the tendency to absorb all of the liquid in the pot. Therefore, when cooking buckwheat, check it frequently, and add more liquid if necessary.

Nutritional content

Buckwheat is low in fat and an excellent source of protein, complex carbohydrates, and both soluble and insoluble fibre. It also contains the antioxidant rutin and provides an array of nutrients, such as manganese, magnesium, thiamin, and riboflavin. Buckwheat is gluten-free, and therefore suitable for those who have coeliac disease or a gluten allergy.

Health benefits

Diets rich in buckwheat are known to lower cholesterol and blood pressure. After studying the Yi people of China, a population that generally consumes 100 grams (3½oz) of buckwheat daily per person, scientists concluded that the consumption of buckwheat lowers total blood cholesterol and bad (Low Density Lipids, or LDL) cholesterol levels while improving the ratio of good (High Density Lipids, or HDL) to bad (LDL) cholesterol.

Diets rich in buckwheat have also been shown to aid in the management of type 2 diabetes. Bread made from buckwheat groats lowers blood glucose levels considerably, and improves the pancreas's insulin response after consumption.

In addition, the magnesium in buckwheat may contribute to lowering the risk of type 2 diabetes by as much as 24 per cent. Magnesium is also known to relax blood vessels, and in doing so, lowers blood pressure and improves the delivery of nutrients to cells.

FACTS

Diets rich in buckwheat are proven to reduce cholesterol and blood pressure.

•

The magnesium in buckwheat may reduce the risk of type 2 diabetes by 24 per cent.

•

Blood glucose levels and insulin response in type 2 diabetics may be better managed by eating buckwheat regularly.

•

A gluten-free food, buckwheat is suitable for those who suffer from coeliac disease or are allergic to gluten.

corn

Easy to grow and protein-rich, corn may be enjoyed boiled whole as a tasty, sweet vegetable, popped as popcorn, or milled into polenta or cornmeal to make irresistible baked goods. Once a staple of Native American tribes, today, the largest amounts of this important crop are grown in the United States, Russia, China, Mexico, and Brazil.

History

Thought to have originated in Central America, corn has served as a staple food for native civilizations in primitive times and continues to hold a central place in the diets of Native American cultures today. Because of their heavy reliance on corn for sustenance, the Mayan, Aztec, and Incan civilizations regarded corn as a sacred food and incorporated it into their mythology and rituals.

Early explorers discovered corn growing all across America in solid, smooth, and striped varieties, as well as a bright array of colours such as blue, pink, yellow, and black. When Spanish and Portuguese explorers returned from the New World, they brought corn home with them, soon spreading corn around Europe and the rest of the world.

Description

Known scientifically as *Zea mays,* but also commonly called maize, corn grows in "ears" that are dotted with rows of kernels and cushioned by silky fibres, or "corn silk". (Sweetcorn is a sweet-tasting variety that is meant to be eaten as a young, or fresh, vegetable.)

The rigid green husk around the ear provides excellent protection from the elements. The original corn of around 5000 BC is thought to have possessed few kernels. After thousands of years of domestication, techniques have been developed for producing plump, kernel-filled ears.

Cornmeal or milled corn, can be used to make anything from breads to pancakes. Usually, corn undergoes a milling process in which the ears are cleaned, steamed, the husks removed, and the corn ground, leaving only the endosperm of the kernel as cornmeal. The cornmeal is then enriched to replace a few of the nutrients lost during milling. It is therefore best to purchase stoneground cornmeal, which is coarsely ground in a way that allows the rich germ inside to remain intact. Avoid "degerminated"

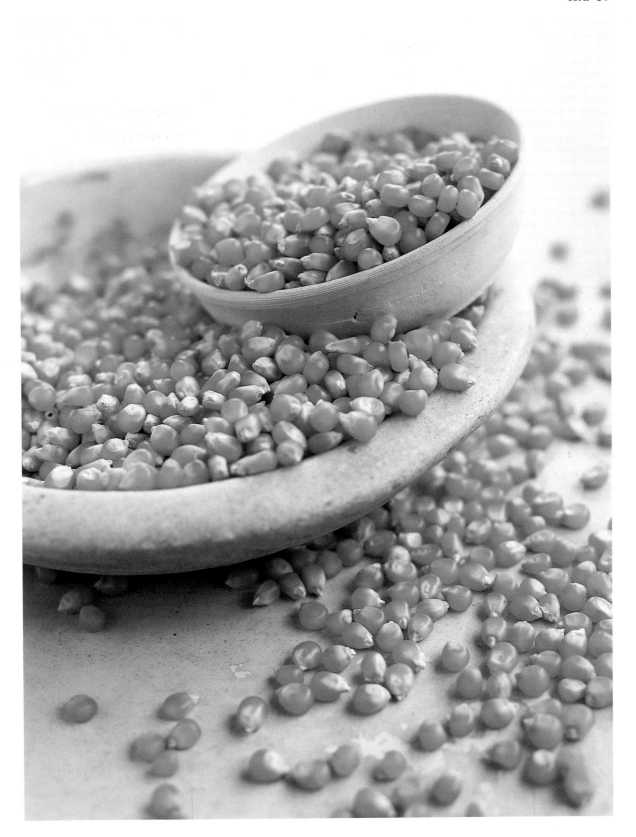

cornmeal which has the germ removed. Cornmeal comes in yellow and white varieties depending on whether it's made from yellow or white corn. For those with gluten allergies, cornmeal products provide wonderful alternatives to wheat as they are gluten-free.

Popcorn was a feature of Native Americans' traditional ceremonies long before explorers landed on American shores. In more recent times, popcorn has stood the test of time as a fun, healthy, and popular snack. It's fat-free, sugar-free, has no artificial additives, and relatively few calories when air-popped.

How exactly does popcorn pop? The starchy bran and germ surround the endosperm, which actually contains some water. When the kernel is heated, the water begins to expand and press on the bran surrounding it. When the bran can't take any more pressure, it explodes and the endosperm bursts, turning the kernel inside out. As the built-up steam flows out, we take out the freshly popped corn and smell that deliciously unmistakable popcorn aroma.

Polenta is a cornmeal mash that originated as a prime source of sustenance for peasants in the Italian countryside. Today, polenta is popular in homes around the world as a tasty, nutritious dish, which can be eaten either on its own or as an accompaniment to other dishes. However, polenta is rarely made from wholemeal corn, and is therefore not a wholegrain source.

Cooking corn

Corn can be boiled or steamed quite easily without its husk, or it can be roasted in the husk. Just take care that you do not overcook the ears, as they may become rigid and lose some of their flavour. If you choose to roast the ears in the husk, be sure to soak them first. One popular method is to open the husk carefully to remove the silk, season with olive oil, salt, and pepper, and then fold back the leaves of husk and roast over a low heat on a grill or barbecue.

Polenta: Making wholegrain polenta from scratch requires time and lots of stirring. Boil 2 litres (3½ pints) of water. As the pot continues to boil, pour in 450 grams (1lb) of coarsely ground whole cornmeal, and stir the mixture. Keep stirring in the same direction for about 20–30 minutes. The more you stir it, the better it will turn out.

Once it has finished cooking, it should have a pudding-like consistency. You can either serve it as it is, or sprinkled with Parmesan cheese, topped with sautéed vegetables, or served alongside chicken, fish, or lean meat.

ADVICE

Choose stoneground cornmeal, which is coarsely ground, leaving the rich germ intact.

●

For a healthy snack that's high in fibre and other nutrients, try making your own popcorn.

●

Boiled, steamed, or roasted corn on the cob makes a healthy and delicious fast-food treat.

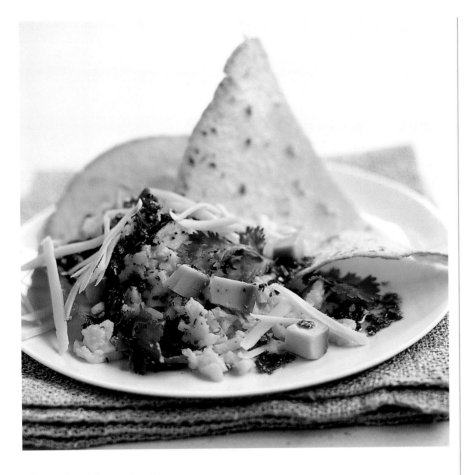

wholegrain corn huevos
rancheros with salsa verde
(*see p85*).

Nutritional content

Corn is considered a starchy vegetable because of its high carbohydrate
content. It also contains an abundance of thiamin, folate, dietary fibre,
vitamin C, phosphorus, and manganese. Corn is low in fat, is a good source
of soluble and insoluble fibre, and is appropriate in the diets of anyone
allergic to gluten.

Health benefits

Corn is a good source of fibre – including both soluble and insoluble.
Soluble fibre helps to stabilize blood sugar levels, and is therefore thought
to reduce the risk of developing type 2 diabetes. The soluble fibre corn
contains may also lower cholesterol levels, contributing to the prevention
of heart disease.

   The insoluble fibre corn provides helps to keep the gastrointestinal tract
in good condition and may reduce the risk of colon cancer. Corn is also an
excellent source of folate, which is believed to contribute to a healthy heart
and may reduce the risk of heart attacks.

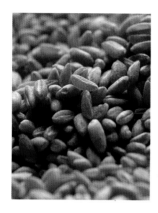

farro

One of the oldest grains in the world, farro was the food of choice for armies in the Roman Empire as it was easy to produce and rich in nutrients. Deriving its name from the Italian word "farina", meaning flour, farro is an ancient relative of spelt and durum wheat. Today, it is a staple crop of Ethiopia and a gourmet ingredient in Italian kitchens.

FACTS

Rich in nutrients, farro is an excellent source of fibre, magnesium, vitamins A, B, C, and E.

•

Farro is an ancient relative of spelt and durum wheat.

•

Low in gluten, but not free from it, farro may be eaten by some people who have a mild sensitivity to gluten.

History

Cultivation of farro, along with wheat and barley, began about 10,000 years ago in the Near and Far East, Europe, and North Africa. Development of farro eventually slowed throughout the Middle Ages as farmers began to favour wheat, barley, and other newly cultivated grains. By 1900, farro was only cultivated in parts of Russia, Italy, Ethiopia, and India.

Description

Farro, and its "cousins" emmer and einkorn, are known as "hulled wheats" meaning the berry or kernel retains its hull during harvest and must be dehulled prior to further processing. The edible portion of the grain grows within the hull, which protects it from environmental damage and contamination from pesticides.

Cooking farro

Rinse farro in cool water and soak it for at least eight hours before cooking. Boil farro in the water used for soaking for approximately two hours. Remove from the heat and allow the grains to sit for several minutes so they can fully absorb any remaining liquid. Well-prepared farro has a texture that is both chewy and firm. To cut cooking time in half, prepare farro in a pressure-cooker.

Nutritional content

Farro is an exceptional source of fibre, magnesium, and vitamins A, B, C, and E. Farro has a low gluten content, which may allow some people who are sensitive to gluten to enjoy the grain.

Health benefits

Farro has yet to be the focus of any major clinical studies, but it is rich in nutrients, and therefore an excellent choice for health and nutrition.

kamut

Kamut earns its name from the Egyptian word for "wheat", which also means "soul of the earth". It is, in fact, an ancient relative of durum wheat and grows to twice the size of common wheat. Kamut is able to thrive without the use of fertilizers and pesticides and is becoming more popular as the demand for organic farming increases worldwide.

History

Legend has it that kamut entered the United States after a US airman discovered the grains hidden within an ancient Egyptian stone box. Bringing back only a handful of kernels, the airman gave them to a friend to farm. The kamut crop was an amusing sight: the plants looked exactly like common wheat, only enormous! The farmer called his plant "King Tut's Wheat" and sold it as a novelty item at fairs. The novelty soon wore off, and it wasn't until the 1980s that there was a resurgence of interest in kamut. It is now cultivated in small areas of the US and Canada.

Description

Although it looks similar to durum wheat, kamut contains 20–40 per cent more protein, fats, vitamins, and minerals. Naturally sweet and buttery in flavour, kamut is delicious in cereals, baked goods, pastas, and breads.

Cooking kamut

To cook kamut, boil one part of the grain in three parts water, adding a dash of salt. The grain will take up to two hours to cook.

Nutritional content

Kamut is an excellent source of protein, essential fatty acids, vitamins, and minerals. It is also a good source of selenium, magnesium, zinc, and vitamin E. Kamut contains gluten and should not be eaten by anyone with a gluten sensitivity or wheat allergy.

Health benefits

As a newly rediscovered grain, kamut has not yet been the focus of many scientific studies. However, with its array of vitamins, minerals, amino acids, and antioxidants, kamut surely offers many of the same health benefits as wholewheat.

FACTS

An ancient relative of durum wheat, kamut contains 20–40 per cent more protein, essential fatty acids, vitamins, and minerals than durum wheat.

•

A newly rediscovered grain, kamut is cultivated without the use of fertilizers and pesticides, and is becoming increasingly popular as the demand for organic farming grows worldwide.

•

Kamut contains gluten and should not be eaten by anyone who is allergic or sensitive to wheat.

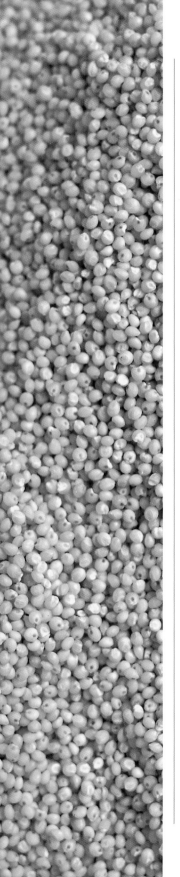

millet

Millet is one of the oldest and most nutritious grains in the world. Originating in the Ethiopian region of Africa in prehistoric times, it was even discussed in the Bible as an ingredient in unleavened bread. Once used primarily as birdseed and livestock fodder in the West, it is now gaining momentum as a healthy grain for our everyday diets.

History

Millet has long been an important food staple in both Africa and India, where it is still used to make the traditional Ethiopian flatbread, *injera*, and the Indian flatbread, *roti*. During the Middle Ages, millet became popular in Eastern Europe, where it was used in the preparation of traditional dishes such as porridge and kasha. Millet was introduced to the United States in the 18th century by settlers from Europe. Today, the main worldwide producers of millet are India, China, and Nigeria.

Description

The term millet may refer to a variety of grains, most of which are used as birdseed and not consumed as food. The millet that you are most likely to see in your local grocery store or health food shop is *Panicum miliaceuem* or *Setaria italica*. There are four major varieties of millet – Pearl, Foxtail, Finger, and Proso millet. Pearl millet is the largest of the four and most frequently used for food products.

Millet looks like a tall grass that is similar to corn. The millet seeds are surrounded by a hard, indigestible hull, so they have to be hulled in order to be used for human consumption. Because the germ remains intact, hulling does not affect the nutrient value of the grain. Millet seeds are small, round, and pearly looking. They come in a variety of colours: yellow, white, grey, or red. Millet is a versatile grain that can grow in many different regions. It grows well in climates with both high and low temperatures, needs little moisture, and has a short growing season.

Cooking millet

You can use millet to make just about anything from cereals, casseroles, and breads to stews, pilafs, and stuffing. You can make it as a side dish by mixing it with vegetables or combining it with a variety of spices and other grains for flavourful salads.

Its tasty, mildly sweet, nut-like quality makes millet ideal for a variety of recipes. Before cooking, wash the millet to remove dirt and sift through to remove any damaged grains. To cook, combine one part millet with three parts boiling water, and cook for about 30 minutes or until you see that the water has been absorbed by the grain. Remove from the heat and leave covered for about 10 more minutes.

If you presoak millet beforehand, cooking time can decrease by 5–10 minutes. If you prefer a fluffier texture, use less water, but if you'd like a dense texture, use more water. To improve millet's flavour, you may wish to roast it in a pan before cooking. Stir it for about three minutes on low heat, or until you detect a nutty, burning aroma. Once you see a golden colour appear, add boiling water and cook as described above. You can, however, experiment with different cooking times and methods if you wish to vary the consistency and flavour of millet.

Millet flour, made by grinding millet, produces light, delicate baked goods. If you wish to use it in yeast breads, use up to 30 per cent and make the rest with gluten-rich flour so the bread will rise. If you want to add a crunch to your baked goods, add raw millet seeds to the flour before baking them.

Millet flakes are millet seeds that have been flattened on a roller. They can be added to muesli or made into porridge for a nutritious breakfast.

Nutritional content

Composed mostly of carbohydrates, millet also has 15 per cent protein, and contains the essential amino acid lysine. It also contains lots of fibre, B vitamins such as niacin, thiamin, and riboflavin, and is a good source of manganese, phosphorous, and magnesium.

Millet does not contain gluten and can be included in a gluten-free diet. It is also an alkaline food, which means it does not form acid, making it quite easy to digest for those who have coeliac disease.

Health benefits

Millet is an incredibly healthy grain, but it is particularly beneficial for the heart. It is rich in the mineral magnesium, which helps to lower blood pressure and may reduce the risk of heart attacks. Magnesium has also been linked to a reduced incidence of migraines and asthma attacks.

Millet also contains phytochemicals such as phytate, which is thought to reduce the risk of cancer, and phytic acid, which may lower cholesterol levels. Foxtail millet has been found to be particularly high in the trace element silicon, which may be beneficial for hair, skin, and nails.

FACTS

The germ remains intact during the hulling process, ensuring the nutrient value of the grain is unaffected.

•

Millet is gluten-free, making it easily digestible for those with coeliac disease.

•

Including millet in your diet is thought to reduce the risk of cancer and lower cholesterol levels.

•

Millet is a good source of protein, and essential nutrients such as B vitamins, manganese, phosphorous, and magnesium.

oats

Oats have been produced and consumed worldwide for several thousand years. Because oats are hardy and can withstand poor soil conditions that may be unsuitable for other grains, they thrive in various regions. Today, the major commercial producers of oats include Russia, Germany, Poland, Finland, and the United States.

History

Although oats have become popular as a nutritious breakfast food, their origins were much more humble. Deriving from the wild red oat plant in Asia, oats are believed to have grown as uncultivated weeds in the presence of other crops. The domestication of oats occurred around 2500 BC, probably in northern Africa, the Near East, and temperate areas of Russia. Before gaining wide acceptance as a food staple, oats were used as animal feed or bedding for livestock. For thousands of years, Europe was the centre of commercial oat production, and oats figured prominently in the diets of people in Scotland, England, Germany, and Scandinavia. Scottish settlers introduced oats to North America in the 17th century.

Description

Oats (*Avena sativa*) undergo special processing after being harvested to provide consumers with a variety of products. Although all oats are hulled, this process does not strip away the bran and germ, allowing oats to retain their exclusive flavour, along with a multitude of nutrients and fibre.

Rolled oats are the most well-known form of oats. Their flat shape results from being hulled, steamed, and then pressed with steel rollers. They puff up quickly when cooked (5–7 minutes) and are easy to chew and digest. They are the preferred type of oats for oatmeal, muesli, and fruit crumbles.

Quick oats are just like rolled oats, except they are sliced thinly before being rolled. This allows them to cook more rapidly (3–5 minutes).

Instant oats are loved by many for their convenience. They are made of groats that have been cut into tiny pieces, then precooked, dried, and rolled very thin. Flavoured varieties generally include sugar, salt, and other ingredients that should be avoided, so read labels carefully.

FACTS

The hulling process leaves the bran and germ intact, allowing oats to retain a multitude of nutrients and fibre.

•

Daily consumption of oats may help to lower cholesterol, boost heart health, maintain a healthy weight, and manage diabetes.

•

Oats are an excellent source of manganese, which helps control blood sugar levels.

•

Oats can trigger symptoms in those with a gluten intolerance or coeliac disease, so avoid them if you suffer from either condition.

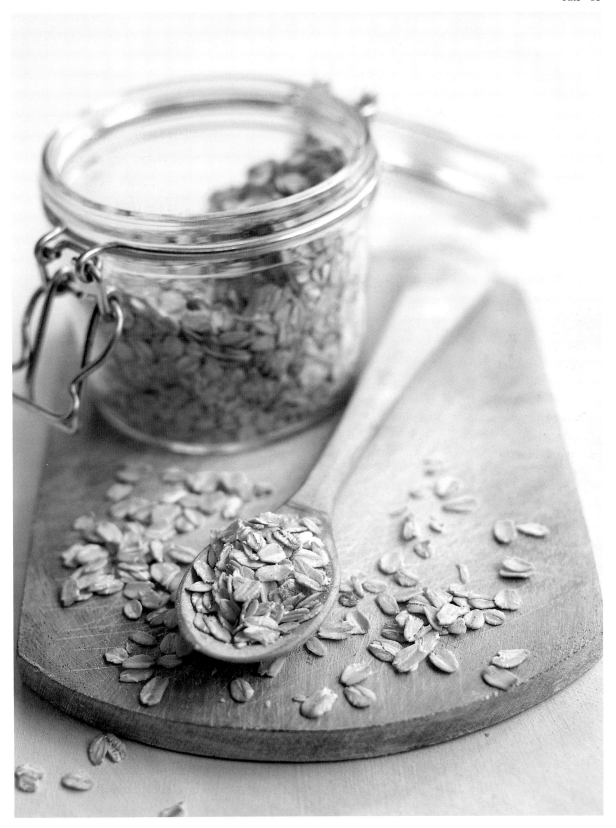

Oat groats (whole oats) involve minimal processing, only removing the hull. Because groats can be difficult to chew, they require more cooking time (about 50 minutes) and more water. They are best for breakfast cereals, hearty breads, and flavourful salads.

Steel-cut oats (Irish oats or Scotch oats) are chewier than rolled oats, and are actually oat groats chopped into small pieces. They are used to make oatmeal porridge.

Oat flour is used in baked goods such as pancakes and muffins and also as a thickening agent in soups and sauces. It is made by grinding groats into a fine powder, and you can produce your own oat flour by grinding rolled oats in a blender, if you wish.

Oat bran is the outer layer of the grain that is removed from the groats during processing. Oat bran can be found in all wholegrain oats, but it can also be purchased separately. While it is not a wholegrain, oat bran is healthy and versatile and can be added to hot and cold cereals, as well as used in muffins, cakes, and breads. However, avoid commercial oat bran muffins, as they can contain more than 500 calories and lots of fat.

Cooking oats

Oats add great taste and texture to any meal, and best of all, they go a long way towards boosting your fibre intake. When buying oats, it is always wise to do so in small quantities because oats have a slightly higher fat content than other grains and may turn rancid more quickly. If you buy a prepared product like instant porridge, look at the nutritional information and select products with the least amount of sugar.

When cooking any kind of oat product, it is best to use twice as much water as oats – that is, two parts water to one part oats. Add the oats to cold water and bring them to the boil. Because oat groats and steel-cut oats are thicker than other oats, they require three parts water to one part groats and should be cooked for a longer period of time.

Oats add great texture, taste, and fibre to any meal. Add oat flour to your favourite baked goods, use them as a topping for fruit crumbles, or try using ground oats as breading for fish or chicken.

Nutritional content

Oats are a good source of complex carbohydrates and fibre, and they contain protein too. They are also a rich source of vitamins and minerals including thiamin, selenium, phosphorus, and manganese. Oats contain

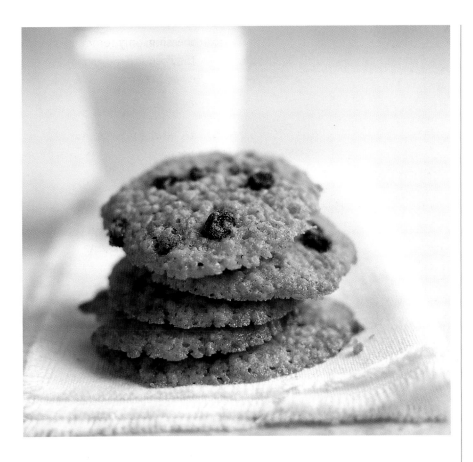

oatmeal raisin cookies
(*see pp150–51*).

smaller amounts of folate, vitamin E, and the minerals copper and zinc. Some quick-cooking oat packets are also enriched with vitamins and minerals, such as iron. Avoid oats if you have a gluten intolerance or coeliac disease, as it can elicit a response in some sufferers.

Health benefits

Eating oats on a daily basis is a great way to maintain a healthy weight or lose weight, lower cholesterol, boost heart health, and prevent or manage type 2 diabetes. The Food and Drug Administration (FDA) in the United States recommends eating oatmeal as part of a low saturated fat, low cholesterol diet, to help reduce the risk of heart disease.

Much of their disease-fighting power comes from the rich amounts of fibre oats contain – nearly 55 per cent soluble fibre and 45 per cent insoluble fibre. In fact, oats contain more soluble fibre than any other grain. Soluble fibre dissolves in water and turns into a viscous gel when digested, which moves very slowly through the intestinal tract. This may explain why eating oats has been shown to reduce the absorption of sugar, or glucose, into the bloodstream, thereby benefiting type 2 diabetics.

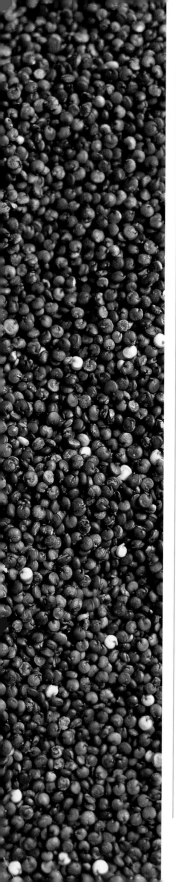

quinoa

Native to the mountains of South America, quinoa (pronounced keen-wah) was the esteemed dietary staple of the ancient Incas. A plant so nourishing and essential to the Inca warriors, it earned the title "the gold of the Incas". Grown in Bolivia, Ecuador, Chile, and the United States, quinoa is thought to be the world's healthiest grain.

History

Championing it for its ability to grow in the poor, arid soil of the Andes, the Incas began cultivating quinoa over 5,000 years ago. The grain was so vital that, when the Spanish Conquistadors invaded, they destroyed the sprawling fields of quinoa, knowing the population relied upon the grain for survival. Additionally, the conquistadors made it illegal for the Incas to grow quinoa, punishing the crime with death. Fortunately, the hardy grain thrived in the Andean soil and survived the Spanish invasion.

In North America, the benefits of quinoa remained virtually unknown until the 1980s. It was only then that farmers, upon learning of quinoa's impressive nutritional content and creamy, light flavour, began cultivating it in the Colorado Rockies, and quinoa has grown in popularity ever since.

Description

Although quinoa is typically classified as a grain, it is, in fact, a vegetable seed. With the scientific name *Chenopodium quino Willd.*, the plant is distantly related to spinach, beetroot, and Swiss chard. The seeds of the plant are small, with a flattened oval shape. Colours range from yellow to red, purple to black. The most widely eaten variety of quinoa is a pale, nearly translucent yellow.

Quinoa pasta is the perfect choice for anyone looking for delicious, gluten-free pasta. It comes in a variety of shapes and is gaining in popularity, becoming increasingly available in health food shops.

Quinoa flour is a tasty, gluten-free alternative to wheat flour. To bake with quinoa flour, substitute the quinoa flour for the refined flour, reducing the given measurements by half. If replacing wholewheat flour, follow the recipe's recommended measurements. Because it has a higher fat content than traditional flour, quinoa produces moist and delicious baked goods.

Quinoa flakes are made from whole quinoa kernels that have been rolled into flat flakes. They make a delicious alternative to porridge oats in hot or cold breakfast cereal. Simply add milk or water and leave to stand for up to three minutes. Add chopped fruits, nuts, and honey for a tasty breakfast. Quinoa flakes are also a delicious addition to soups, stews, and casseroles.

Cooking quinoa

Before cooking quinoa, rinse it thoroughly under cool water to remove the saponin, a soaplike layer that has a bitter flavour and can potentially irritate the digestive tract. After rinsing, combine one part quinoa with two parts water and bring to the boil. Once the mixture boils, reduce the heat, cover, and simmer until the water is absorbed. Quinoa normally cooks within 10 minutes. Before serving, allow the quinoa to steam for five minutes and then fluff with a fork.

Instead of white rice, use quinoa to prepare your favourite rice dishes such as stir-fries and pilafs. Quinoa also makes a delicious addition to salads and stuffings.

Nutritional content

Quinoa is an excellent source of carbohydrates, as well as high-quality protein. About 13–14 per cent of quinoa's total calories come from protein, and it also contains all of the essential amino acids, including lysine, methionine, and cystine.

In addition, quinoa is low in fat, high in fibre, and is a good source of B vitamins and minerals such as iron, magnesium, calcium, and potassium. Quinoa is also a gluten-free wholegrain, which makes it a suitable food for people who suffer from coeliac disease.

Health benefits

Purported to be the most nutritious grain in the world, quinoa has the ability to improve health from head to toe. For anyone who suffers from migraines, incorporating quinoa into the diet is a wise decision. The magnesium found in quinoa relaxes blood vessels, which may reduce the frequency of migraine headaches. Eating quinoa has also been found to improve energy metabolism in brain and muscle cells, and this may lead to fewer headaches.

The high fibre content of quinoa has been shown to lower cholesterol and blood pressure. In addition, the fibre it contains may reduce the risk of gallstone formation and heart disease. In short, quinoa is one of the world's most nutritionally perfect foods, and introducing it into your diet is a smart and tasty choice.

FACTS

Quinoa is low in fat and high in fibre. Adding quinoa to your diet may help to lower cholesterol and blood pressure, and reduce the risk of heart disease.

•

An excellent source of complete protein, the World Health Organisation has rated the quality of protein in quinoa as at least equivalent to that in milk.

•

Rich in magnesium, quinoa may help to reduce the frequency of migraine headaches.

rice

For much of the world, rice is the essence of the daily diet. Cultivated more than 6,000 years ago in Asia, rice is both a cultural and nutritional staple across the world. Rice thrives in warm, humid climates, and is so pervasive that, in many languages, the verb "to eat" is derived from the phrase "to eat rice".

FACTS

The fibre and selenium in brown rice may help to prevent colon cancer.

•

Eating brown rice helps to lower cholesterol levels and maintain stable blood sugar levels.

•

One serving of brown rice provides 88 per cent of the recommended daily amount of manganese, which helps control blood sugar levels.

•

Rice is gluten-free and is ideal for people with a gluten intolerance.

History

An ancient Chinese religious ceremony centred upon the Emperor's sowing of the annual rice, marking the significance of rice in the ancient world. In many countries rice still holds ceremonial significance, it symbolizes fertility and is thrown at weddings to wish fertility upon the bride and groom. Buddhism carried rice throughout Asia, ensuring the nutritional, religious, and political importance of rice across the continent. After their invasion of India, the armies of Alexander the Great brought rice to Europe. By the 17th century, rice was cultivated in Africa, Asia, Europe, and North America. With nearly 200 billion pounds produced each year, the popularity of rice is assured.

Description

Unfortunately, much of the rice produced each year goes through a complicated machine-milling process to produce white rice. The discarded bran and germ layers contain much of the kernel's fibre, protein, vitamins, and minerals, leaving behind only the endosperm, which makes up 75 per cent of the rice kernel and consists of mostly starch.

The purest form of rice is wholegrain brown rice (*Oryza Sativa*), in which only the inedible husk is removed. Although brown rice is the most common wholegrain rice, there are also red, black, and purple varieties.

Long-grain brown rice is common in Indian and Western cuisine and maintains a firm texture after cooking. Because it is the least starchy of the rice varieties, long-grain rice does not stick together when cooked.

Medium-grain brown rice is a softer and plumper variety than long-grain, and is used in cereals and rice cakes. It is also common in Latin and Asian dishes and is often used in soups and side dishes.

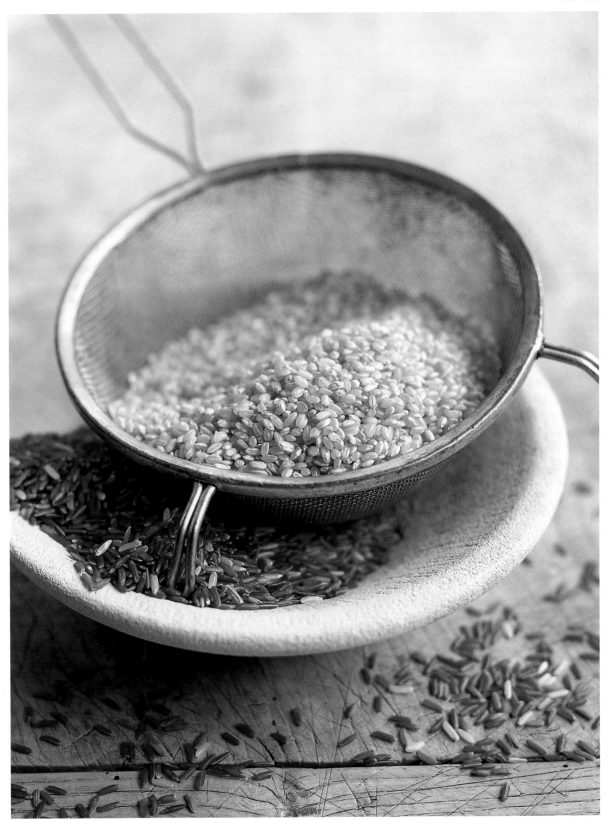

Short-grain brown rice, also known as "sticky rice", is an integral part of Japanese cooking, including sushi. However, these meals are often prepared with white rice, which has been processed and contains few nutrients. Ask for brown rice when dining in restaurants, and prepare meals with brown rice at home.

Sweet brown rice or "mochi rice" is eaten primarily in Japan as part of sushi or dessert, and is a high-protein, quick-cooking variety. This very sticky rice is nearly translucent when cooked, but, again, is primarily sold as white rice.

Aromatic rice such as Indian Basmati and Thai Jasmine are available in brown wholegrain forms. Basmati rice, cultivated in the Himalayas, is a long-grain variety with a mild, nutty flavour. Jasmine rice has a sweet and delicate flavour named after its renowned Jasmine fragrance.

Quick-cooking brown rice is a precooked variety of brown rice, designed for convenience because it cooks quickly. New varieties of brown rice are now available that cook in only a few minutes.

Wild rice (*Zizania aquatica*) is an entirely separate species to brown rice, and despite its name, is not actually rice at all. A member of the grass family, wild rice flourishes without cultivation on the banks of North American wetlands. Because the plant grows wild, 60 per cent of the annual crop is lost, making wild rice a speciality food.

Cooking rice

To cook brown rice, pour one part rice into two parts boiling water or broth. After the liquid returns to the boil, lower the temperature, cover, and simmer for 35–45 minutes. Be sure to cook rice in an amount of water that can be fully absorbed by the rice. If cooked in excess liquid and drained, vital nutrients will be lost with the discarded liquid.

Nutritional content

An excellent source of carbohydrates, manganese, selenium, phosphorus, magnesium, and B vitamins, rice is truly a nutritional powerhouse. However, the milling and polishing process that converts brown rice to white rice removes the majority of these essential nutrients. Also, because brown rice retains its bran layer, it contains four times more insoluble fibre than white rice. Rice is gluten-free and one of the most easily digested grains, making it ideal for those with a gluten intolerance.

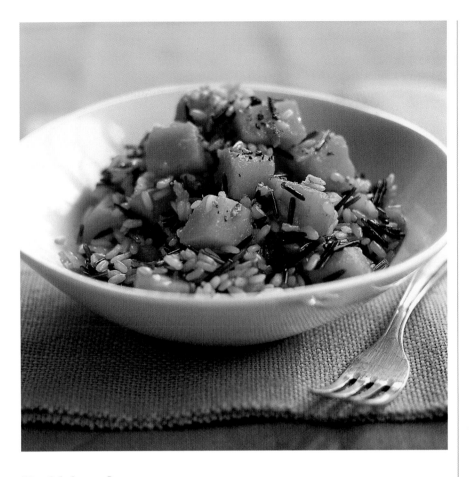

curried squash risotto with
brown and wild rice
(*see pp140–41*).

Health benefits

The scientifically proven benefits of rice have far-reaching effects
on health. One serving of brown rice contains 88 per cent of the
recommended daily amount of manganese, which helps to control
blood sugar levels.

Because of its combination of insoluble fibre and selenium, eating
brown rice on a regular basis may help prevent colon cancer. Insoluble
fibre minimizes the amount of time that carcinogenic materials spend
in contact with colon cells, while selenium has been shown to inhibit
the propagation of cancer cells.

For people with elevated cholesterol levels, incorporating brown rice
into the diet is a wise decision. The oil in the bran of whole brown rice has
been shown to lower LDL ("bad") cholesterol. Additionally, brown rice
raises blood levels of nitric acid, a molecule known to impede development
of plaque in the arteries. The fibre found in brown rice has also been shown
to lower cholesterol levels. Finally, the fibre in brown rice helps the body to
maintain stable blood sugar levels, and prevents gallstone formation.

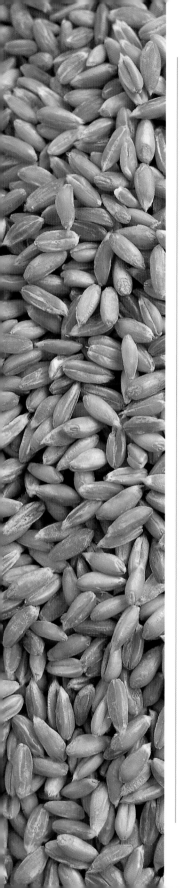

rye

Ground mostly into flour for bread, rye is a staple in many countries in Northern Europe. Rye is also delicious eaten whole, as an alternative to rice, or as rye flakes for a tasty breakfast cereal. Rye can grow in areas too cold or wet for other grains to survive – it is mainly cultivated in Russia, Canada, Poland, Germany, and Denmark.

History

German farmers first considered rye to be just a pesky weed growing among the wheat and barley crops. Fortunately, it was not long before they discovered that this stubborn weed, flourishing in the harsh northern climate, had a unique and appealing flavour. Eastern European and Scandinavian countries soon incorporated rye into their daily diets. In Finland, rye bread is baked into a flattened disk shape with a hole in the middle. This traditional shape harks back to a time when breads were strung on horizontal poles beneath farmhouse ceilings for storage. In Germany, traditional rye bread became so common that the word for supper, *abendbrot,* is literally translated to mean "evening bread".

Description

Known scientifically as *Secale cereale,* rye bears a slight resemblance to wheat in appearance. Cultivated in varieties ranging from green to brown to yellow, rye is generally found in whole or cracked form. Although it contains gluten, rye's gluten differs from wheat's in that it undergoes a different leavening process, producing more elastic, dense dough. The result is baked goods with a moist, compact, and hearty texture.

When buying rye bread, read ingredient labels carefully to ensure that you are buying bread made of whole rye flour, not a product made of refined flour and coloured with molasses to resemble true rye bread.

Rye berries or whole rye grains are rye in its purest form. Rye berries may be eaten as a cooked cereal or added to flours and multigrain pilaf.

Rye flour comes in light, medium, and dark varieties. Unlike some other grains, the germ and bran of the rye grains are firmly attached to the endosperm so that even after the milling process, rye flour retains its germ and bran, resulting in a hardy, nourishing flour.

Rye flakes are rolled whole grains of rye and resemble rolled oats. They can be eaten as a hot morning cereal, similar to porridge, or added to muesli. Rye flakes can also be added to flour in bread recipes, or sprinkled on top for decoration.

Pumpernickel is a dense German sourdough bread made from a mixture of rye flour and coarsely ground rye meal. The bread also contains molasses, which accounts for the bread's dark colour. Choose carefully to ensure the pumpernickel you purchase is made from wholegrain rye flour and rye meal.

Cooking rye

Before boiling, rinse whole rye under cool, running water. Boil one part rye in four parts water. Add a pinch of salt and let the combination return to a boil. Reduce the heat, leaving it to simmer for one hour. For softer grains, soak the rye overnight and cook it in the soaking water for several hours. For a tasty side dish, sauté the cooked berries in a little olive oil and serve as an alternative to rice.

Substitute rye flour for wheat flour in any of your favourite recipes. Instead of buying crackers made from refined white flour, look for those made from rye.

Nutritional content

Rye is an excellent source of manganese, which is essential for many enzymes to do their job in the body. In addition, rye is a good source of fibre, selenium, phosphorus, magnesium, and protein. Rye contains gluten and is therefore not recommended for those with a gluten intolerance.

Health benefits

Studies show that rye bread is a smarter choice for diabetics than wholewheat bread because it does not induce the same insulin response that wholewheat bread does. Research suggests it is not the fibre of rye bread that leads to stabilized blood sugar levels, but perhaps the dense starch granules of rye. Scientists hypothesize that these dense starch granules, forming a thick matrix, slow the digestion of bread. Slowed digestion leads to a lengthened transformation of starch into sugar, which accounts for steady insulin levels.

For menopausal women, a component of the rye grain may reduce the hot flushes and discomfort associated with reduced levels of oestrogen. This is because rye contains a phytoestrogen, a chemical that resembles natural oestrogen and mimics its behaviour in the body.

FACTS

Rye bread is an excellent choice for diabetics as it stabilizes blood sugar levels.

For menopausal women, eating rye may ease hot flushes and other symptoms associated with menopause.

Even after the milling process, rye flour retains its germ and bran, ensuring the essential nutrients are retained.

Rye contains gluten and is therefore not recommended for people with coeliac disease or who have a gluten intolerance.

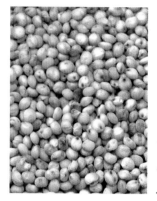

sorghum

Commonly known as "milo", sorghum has been a staple crop in Asia and Africa for centuries. This tropical grass was first domesticated in Ethiopia around 6,000 years ago. Today, sorghum is the fifth most popular grain in the world, and millions of people worldwide benefit from the dazzling array of nutrients it has to offer.

History

Farmers in Africa and India have relied on sorghum for centuries. In the 19th century, sorghum gained notoriety in the Western world in the form of a syrup sweetener. Cheaper to produce than sugar cane, "sorghum molasses" became extremely popular. In fact, it was not until the end of the First World War, when it became less expensive to mass-produce refined sugar, that sorghum fell out of favour.

Description

Able to withstand drought, the sorghum plant flourishes in harsh climates throughout the world. Although it may be difficult to find in traditional supermarkets, speciality shops that carry African and Indian foods often sell a variety of sorghum products, including porridge, breads, and beer.

Cooking sorghum

Sorghum flour is slightly bland, making it the perfect flour to combine with other grains. You can easily make gluten-free pizza crusts, breads, and baked goods with sorghum flour. In addition, whole sorghum grains make a perfect substitute for rice or pasta. Boil one part sorghum in two parts water and bring to a simmer for about 35–40 minutes.

Nutritional content

Sorghum is as nutritious as other grains because it is high in fibre, and contains calcium, potassium, phosphorus, iron, and niacin. In addition to carbohydrates, it also contains protein and a small amount of fat.

Health benefits

Scientific evidence shows that sorghum is closer in its genetic makeup to corn than it is to wheat. Therefore, sorghum is free of gluten and is safe to eat if you have a gluten intolerance or coeliac disease.

spelt

Although the exact origins of spelt are somewhat mysterious, the cultivation of the grain in Europe and the Middle East can be traced back 5,000 years. Nutty and sweet in flavour, and with a lighter texture than other wholegrains, spelt became an indispensable favourite among Germans, Swiss, and Austrians.

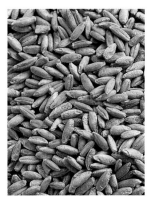

History

Spelt was very important in ancient times, and is mentioned in the Bible as one of the seven original grains. Ancient Roman leaders distributed spelt to the poor as part of the world's first known welfare system. As populations migrated throughout Europe, they introduced spelt to new regions.

Description

Spelt (*Triticum spelta*), a hybrid of emmer and einkorn wheats, combines their best qualities and, in some ways, even exceeds them. Unlike wheat, spelt retains its sturdy outer husk, protecting the grain from pollutants. The husk also helps spelt to retain its nutrients and freshness.

Cooking spelt

Because spelt is low in gluten, products made with spelt flour do not always rise evenly when baking. Experiment with the amount of liquid used in the recipe or mix spelt flour with gluten-rich flour to obtain better results. To cook spelt berries, first soak overnight. Drain. Boil one part spelt in three parts water. Bring to a simmer and cook for about one hour.

Nutritional content

Spelt is an excellent source of fibre and B vitamins, and has 10–25 per cent more protein than wheat. Spelt contains a small amount of gluten and is not appropriate for those with coeliac disease or gluten intolerance.

Health benefits

Spelt is an excellent source of riboflavin, a vitamin necessary for proper energy metabolism within cells. Riboflavin may reduce the frequency of migraines by restoring proper energy metabolism in nervous system cells. Spelt's high soluble fibre content accounts for its positive effects on lowering blood cholesterol levels.

FACTS

Spelt is a nutritional powerhouse – it's an excellent source of fibre, B vitamins, and protein.

•

Eating spelt may reduce the frequency of migraines due to its high riboflavin content.

•

Spelt's high soluble fibre content lowers blood cholesterol levels and improves the ratio of "bad" (LDL) to "good" (HDL) cholesterol.

•

The organic farming movement has embraced the cultivation of spelt as it is more hardy than other varieties of wheat and does not require fertilizer.

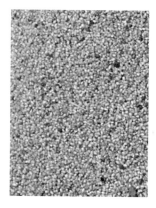

teff

A tiny grain that is jam-packed with nutrients, teff is actually the smallest grain in the world, requiring 150 grains to equal the weight of one grain of wheat. Teff earned its name from the Ethiopian Amharic word for "lost" because its small size made it very difficult for farmers to collect during harvest.

FACTS

Comprised mostly of the nutritious bran and germ, teff is high in protein, fibre, and a range of vitamins and minerals.

•

Including fibre-rich teff in your daily diet may reduce the incidence of type 2 diabetes.

•

As teff is gluten-free, it is suitable for those suffering from coeliac disease and gluten intolerance.

•

Uncooked teff can be eaten as an alternative to nuts or sesame seeds. Add teff to pancake, porridge, or bread recipes for extra flavour and fibre.

History
First cultivated in Ethiopia between 4000 and 1000 BC, teff remains a dietary staple in that region. *Injera*, an Ethiopian bread made from fermented teff, is eaten throughout the country. Teff has only recently made its way to Europe and North America, but it is gaining in popularity and becoming more available in health food and speciality shops.

Description
Teff is a grass that flourishes in both arid conditions and flooded regions. Variations of teff range in colour from white to deep red, brown, or purple. White varieties impart a mild, nutty flavour similar to chestnuts, while darker varieties have a heartier flavour, akin to that of hazelnuts.

Cooking teff
To prepare teff, boil three parts water to one part teff. Reduce the heat, cover, and simmer for 15–20 minutes or until all the water is absorbed. Remove from the heat and leave to stand in a covered pot for 5 minutes.

Nutritional content
As it is so small, the bulk of the teff grain is made up of the nutritious bran and germ. Teff is therefore high in fibre, calcium, phosphorus, iron, copper, and thiamin. Its protein is of exceptional quality, with higher lysine (an amino acid) levels than both wheat and barley. Teff is also low in fat and gluten-free, making it a good choice for people with coeliac disease.

Health benefits
Because of its high fibre content, researchers believe that teff stabilizes blood glucose levels more effectively than other grains. The findings of a recent study suggest that a diet rich in teff (when compared to the typical Western diet) may be linked to a reduced incidence of type 2 diabetes.

triticale

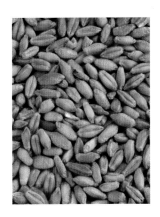

A cross between wheat and rye, triticale was first produced commercially only 80 years ago. Today, there are 6 million acres of triticale grown worldwide. China, France, Poland, and Germany produce 90 per cent of the world's triticale supply, and this wonder grain is slowly, but surely, gaining in popularity.

History

This wheat-rye cross was born out of the need for a high-protein grain that thrives in areas where wheat crops had failed. Triticale combines rye's rugged ability to grow in adverse conditions with wheat's high-protein content and disease resistance. Researchers named this "miracle grain" after the scientific names of its parents: wheat (*Triticum*) and rye (*Secale*).

Description

Triticale is typically sold as flour, berries, and flakes. Triticale flour can make a good substitute for wheat flour. When using triticale flour in a bread recipe, however, knead the dough lightly and allow it to rise only once so as not to interrupt the fermentation process. Boiled triticale flakes make a delicious breakfast cereal, while rich and savoury triticale berries (*see below*) are perfect as a side dish or integrated into a main course.

Cooking triticale berries

Add one part berries to six parts cold water and soak overnight. When you are ready to cook, add 240ml (8fl oz) water and bring to a boil. Allow the berries to simmer for 45–60 minutes. If you wish, after cooking, you can refrigerate the berries for 24 hours before serving.

Nutritional content

Triticale combines the nutritional highlights of its parent grains, wheat and rye. The grain is low in fat, high in fibre, and is a good source of carbohydrates and protein. Triticale does, however, contain gluten.

Health benefits

Triticale has not yet been featured in any major nutritional studies. However, its rich array of nutrients, high fibre content, and similarity to wheat and rye make including triticale in your diet a smart health decision.

FACTS

Triticale is a hardy, high-protein cross between rye and wheat.

•

A versatile grain growing in popularity, look for triticale in speciality and health food shops in the form of flour, berries, and flakes.

•

The gluten in triticale is more delicate than that of wheat. When making bread, knead the dough lightly and allow to rise once for delicious bread.

•

Because triticale contains gluten, it is not recommended for people with coeliac disease or gluten intolerance.

wheat

It is difficult to imagine a world without wheat. It competes with barley as being the oldest cultivated cereal grain. Widely hailed as the most important grain in the world, wheat is essential to the daily diets of people around the globe, and is renowned as the "staff of life". Eat wholewheat rather than refined wheat to reap the nutritional benefits.

History

First cultivated in Western Asia between 8,000 and 10,000 years ago, wheat was largely responsible for mankind's transition from hunter-gatherers to stationary farmers. Anthropologists believe that early man first chewed raw wheat kernels, eventually learning to pound the kernels into flour and mix it with water to make porridge. Ancient Greeks, Romans, and Sumerians demonstrated the importance of wheat in their cultures by worshipping gods and goddesses of wheat. In China, ceremonies celebrating wheat date back to at least 2800 BC. The Egyptians prepared the world's first bread from wheat and barley nearly 6,000 years ago. Baked in clay ovens, the bread became the foundation of the ancient Egyptian diet.

Description

The different species of wheat can be divided into hard and soft varieties. Hard wheat provides fine flour that is ideal for baking breads. The high protein content (12–18 per cent) allows hard wheat flour to absorb a significant amount of water, swelling the dough. On the contrary, soft wheat varieties contain less protein (8–11 per cent), making their flours suitable for the production of cakes, biscuits, crackers, and cereals.

Durum wheat flour is easily distinguished by its amber-coloured kernel and large size. It is the hardiest of all wheat varieties, with a high protein (14–16 per cent) and gluten content, which makes it ideal for the production of firm, high-quality pasta products. When durum is milled, the endosperm is coarsely ground into semolina, a granular, golden-coloured wheat. Because the milling process robs semolina of its nutrient-rich germ and bran, the flour is enriched with some of the nutrients that have been removed – primarily thiamin, riboflavin, niacin, and folate. Fortunately, many pasta makers are now using whole durum flour to make delicious, nutrient-rich wholewheat pasta.

FACTS

Eating wheat bran may reduce the symptoms of diverticulitis and constipation, and has been linked to a decreased risk of breast and colon cancer.

•

Low in fat, wheat contains many essential amino acids, and is an excellent source of dietary fibre.

•

Wheat species are divided into hard and soft varieties. Hard wheat provides fine flour, perfect for breads. Soft wheat flours contain less protein and are good for baking cakes and biscuits.

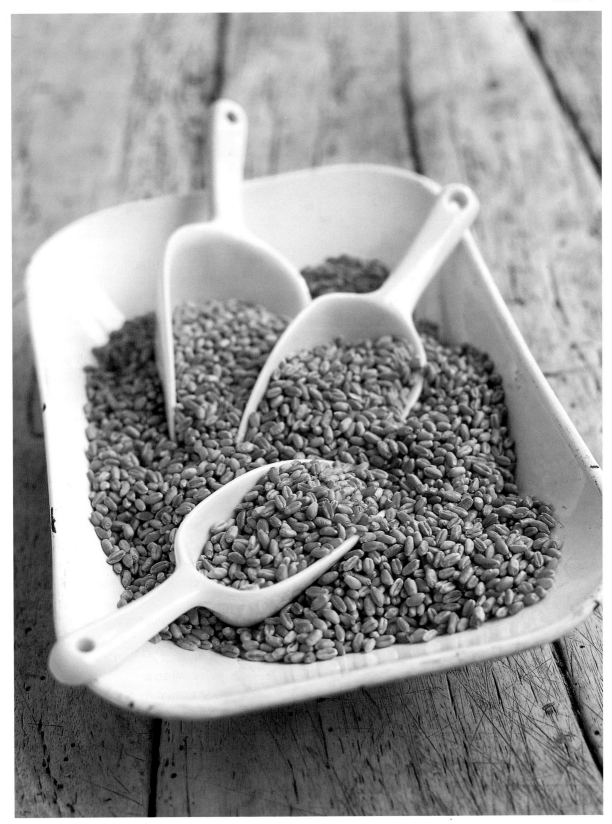

Wholewheat flour is made by grinding the entire wheat kernel into a fine powder. Since the germ and the bran remain, none of the vitamins, minerals, or fibre are lost in processing. Varieties of wholewheat flours include wholewheat baking flour and stoneground wholewheat flour. Quite similar in their nutritional value, these flours are virtually synonymous.

Be careful when purchasing wholewheat flour: "enriched", "unbleached", and "wheat flour" do not mean wholewheat flour. When buying products made from wheat, look for "wholegrain wheat" as the first ingredient listed.

Wheat berries are the dry, one-seeded fruit of wheat, also known as wheat kernels. The purest form of wheat, wheat berries are hard and vary in colour from white to red or purple. Wheat berries make a delicious addition to salads and side dishes.

Bulgur wheat is precooked wheat, made by boiling the wheat kernel and then drying and cracking it into pieces – thus, a minor portion of the coarse outer bran is lost. This is a quick-cooking form of wholewheat with a rich, nut-like flavour and golden colour. Bulgur wheat makes a great dish on its own, or as a side dish. It comes in three varieties: coarse, medium, and fine. Coarse bulgur is generally cooked like rice and used in pilafs and casseroles; medium bulgur is often used as a breakfast cereal; while fine bulgur is an important ingredient in dishes such as tabbouleh, a classic Middle Eastern salad.

Cracked wheat is often confused with bulgur wheat, but is actually made up of raw wholewheat berries that have been ground into coarse granules. Cracked wheat is not precooked like bulgur wheat and has a milder flavour. It is available in fine, medium, and coarse varieties, and is often used in pilafs and salads.

Cooking wheat

Tips on substituting white flour for nutrient-rich, wholewheat flour are described in detail on pages 78–79.

When cooking with wheat berries, it is important to rinse them first. Once clean, boil one part wheat berries in three parts water. Because wheat is so absorbent, one measure of raw berries will yield twice the amount of plump, cooked berries. To halve cooking time, soak the wheat berries overnight in the water you intend to cook them in. Wheat berries should be cooked for roughly 25 minutes if presoaked or 45 minutes if they have not been presoaked. To save even more time, place one part berries in two parts water and microwave on high for 15–18 minutes.

ADVICE

For impressive health benefits, replace refined, white flour with wholewheat flour when making breads, muffins, and even pizza crusts (*for tips, see pp78–79*).

●

When buying wheat products such as rolls, muffins, and crackers, look for "wholegrain wheat" as the first ingredient listed. Choose pasta made from whole durum wheat.

●

To save time when cooking wheat berries, place one part berries in two parts water and microwave on high for 15–18 minutes.

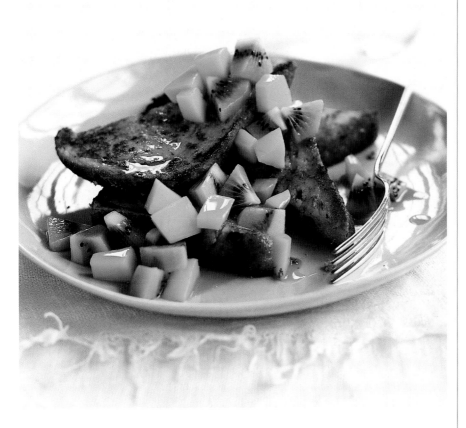

wholegrain French toast
with mango-kiwi fruit salsa
(*see p90*).

Nutritional benefits

Wholewheat contains carbohydrates and boasts an array of nutrients including calcium, iron, B vitamins, magnesium, and phosphorus. It is low in fat, contains many essential amino acids, and is an excellent source of dietary fibre. Wheat contains gluten and is not suitable for people with coeliac disease or gluten allergies.

Health benefits

For anyone familiar with the pains of constipation, wheat bran may be the cure. Studies suggest that adding just 75 grams (2½oz) of wheat bran to your diet per day will significantly reduce the symptoms of diverticulitis and chronic constipation. Wheat bran is also thought to be beneficial in the prevention of colon cancer. Researchers believe that wheat bran reduces the concentration of the bacterial enzymes and bile acids in the faeces that are thought to promote colon cancer. Another recent study found that the insoluble fibre in wheat bran lowers blood oestrogen levels, which may be linked to a decreased risk of breast cancer.

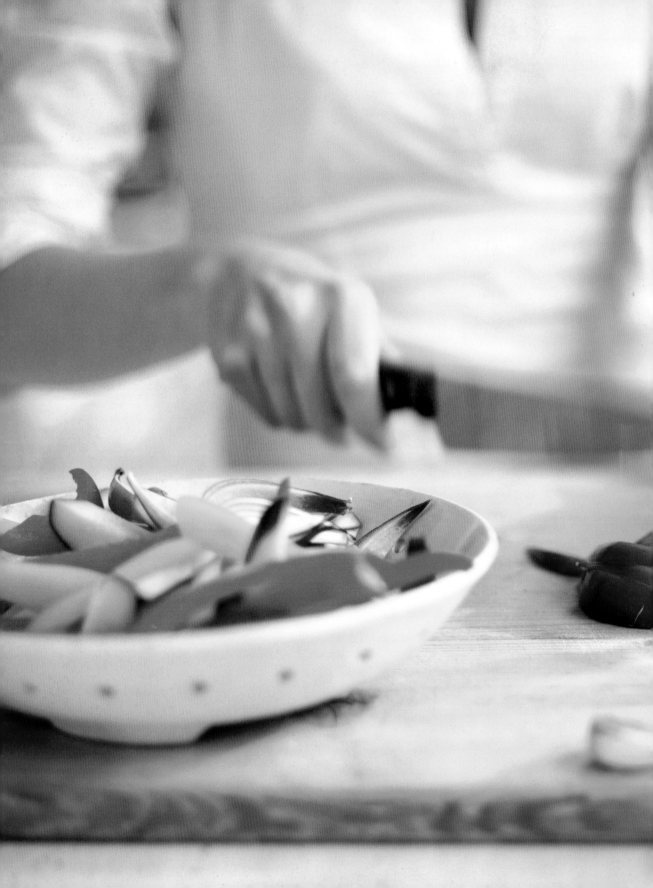

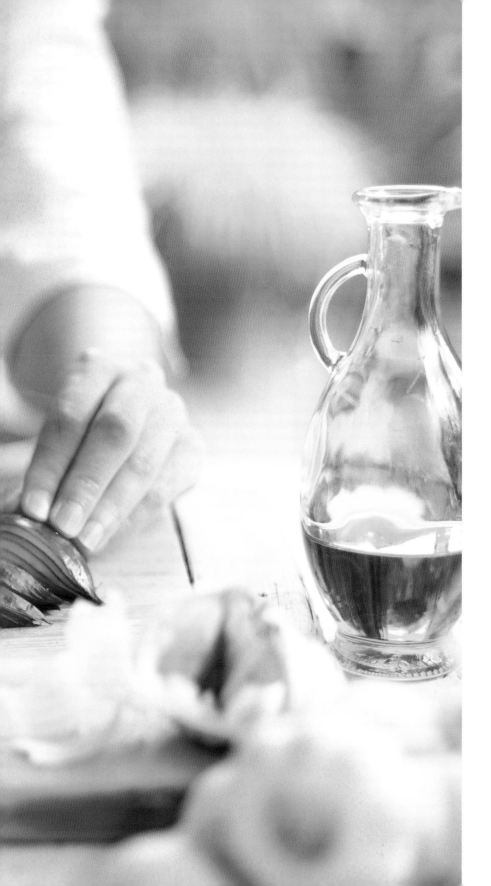

the diet

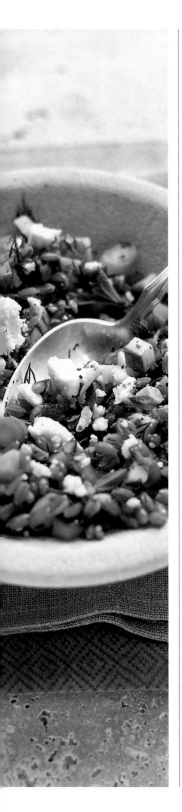

about the diet

If you're like most people living in developed countries, you're probably eating less than one serving of wholegrains every day. We know it can seem daunting to eat three – or more – servings of wholegrains daily (as recommended by nutrition experts) but this four-week diet plan demonstrates how. Showcasing a variety of wholegrain recipes, the diet plan shows you how to achieve lasting, sustainable weight loss. Here are some rules and tips to guide you over the next four weeks.

Drink plenty of water and avoid caffeine
Adding fibre to your diet in the form of wholegrains adds bulk to your stool, which can help keep your bowel movements regular. However, remember to drink six to eight glasses of water a day to prevent bloating and constipation. Limit caffeinated drinks such as tea and coffee – drink decaffeinated versions or herbal tea instead, and if you add milk, use skimmed. Only drink fruit and vegetable juices on the prescribed days.

Limit alcohol intake
No alcohol is to be consumed during the first two weeks of the diet plan. During the last two weeks, limit alcohol to one drink per day. One drink is a 330ml (11½fl oz) beer, 175ml (6 fl oz) glass of wine, or 30ml (1fl oz) spirit with a low-calorie or diet mixer.

Eat on a schedule
Try to eat at similar times of the day. This will help to keep your blood sugar levels steady and your hunger at bay. Also, try to eat slowly, and take the time to enjoy your meals and snacks.

Healthy cooking tips
Always trim the fat from meats before cooking and use a vegetable oil cooking spray and non-stick pans to reduce the need for extra calories. Season food with herbs and spices rather than salt to reduce sodium intake.

Multivitamins and calcium
Take a multivitamin supplement every day to ensure you are getting all the nutrients your body needs. Aim to drink skimmed milk every day (or calcium-enriched lactose-free or soya milk) to ensure you are getting enough calcium.

Exercise regularly

Make three hours of exercise a week your goal. Based on what you do now, start slowly and increase gradually. Begin by walking more often and taking the stairs whenever possible.

Eating out

When dining at restaurants, you don't have to eat the whole portion you are served – eat only until you are satisfied rather than full. See pages 154–55 for more tips on eating wholegrains when dining out.

Vegetarian cooking

Feel free to replace any meat in the recipes or diet plan with the same amount of non-meat proteins such as tofu or TVP (texturized vegetable protein). And, likewise, if you find that you can't find a particular meat or fish for a certain recipe, you may replace it with a comparable protein source.

Keep it simple

Our recipes are easy to prepare and we've tried to keep them as simple as possible. If you don't want to cook every day, swap days around to better accommodate your lifestyle, eating leftovers the following day. (Remember that many of the recipes can be prepared in advance or frozen.) If you're short on time or resources, just stick to the principles of the diet and substitute quick, basic meals for recipes. For example, whip up a vegetable stir-fry and add to it 30g (1oz) of a lean protein source (such as skinless chicken or tofu) and 30g (1oz) of your favourite grain. Alternatively, top 125g (4½oz) wholegrain pasta with a tomato sauce, a protein source, and vegetables.

If any ingredients seem daunting or are difficult to obtain, you can substitute them for something similar, for example, use a vegetable oil cooking spray in place of the various different oils listed, or replace a more unusual grain with an alternative grain (suggested in the recipes).

For better health without following the diet plan

If you want to benefit from eating wholegrains, but don't need to lose weight, aim to eat the recommended three servings per day. Look for small ways to add more wholegrains to your diet, such as swapping regular salad croutons for wholewheat ones, or replacing plain white flour with wholegrain flours in recipes. But don't go overboard when introducing wholegrains, or you'll be adding too many calories. You may gain weight if you top off meals with wholegrain cookies, when you don't usually indulge. Pay close attention to the serving sizes in all our recipes, and if you typically snack between meals, swap refined snacks for wholegrain ones.

ADVICE

Drink at least six to eight glasses of water every day.

•

During the first two weeks of the diet plan, no alcohol is allowed.

•

For weeks 3 and 4 of the diet plan, you can drink one alcoholic beverage per day.

•

Aim to exercise for at least three hours a week.

•

Limit salt intake – cook with fresh or dried herbs rather than salt.

•

Use a non-stick vegetable oil cooking spray and non-stick pans when cooking to reduce the need for extra calories.

•

If not following the diet plan, aim to swap your typical refined snacks for wholegrain ones.

week 1

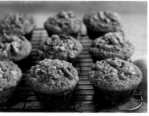 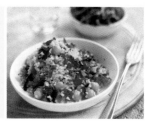

	monday	tuesday	wednesday
breakfast	Banana-walnut oat bran muffin (*see pp88–89*) with 1 tsp low-fat margarine; 240ml (8fl oz) skimmed milk	225g (8oz) oatmeal porridge made with skimmed milk and 2 tbsp raisins	1 wholegrain breakfast bar; ½ grapefruit; 100g (3½oz) low-fat yoghurt
snack	200g (7oz) low-fat yoghurt; 2 tbsp raisins	1 apple; 2 tbsp unsalted nuts	60g (2½oz) low-sugar wholegrain cereal with 240ml (8fl oz) skimmed milk
lunch	1 serving Courgette, barley, and mushroom soup (*see p91*); 6 wholegrain crackers	1 Quinoa tuna salad sandwich on low-calorie wholemeal bread (*see p111*) with 1 sliced tomato and 1 tbsp low-fat mayonnaise	1 serving Lemon bulgur salad with chickpeas and roasted peppers (*see pp104–105*); garden salad with 2 tbsp low-fat dressing
dinner	170g (6oz) grilled salmon; 150g (5½oz) brown rice; steamed string beans with almonds; garden salad with 2 tbsp low-fat dressing	1 serving Red kidney beans and spelt (*see p122*); steamed green and red peppers	170g (6oz) grilled fish with onion, pepper, and tomato salad; 1 serving Millet mashers (*see p131*); steamed spinach
dessert or snack	3 kiwi fruit	1 sliced cantaloupe melon	125g (4½oz) fresh berries with 100g (3½oz) low-fat yoghurt

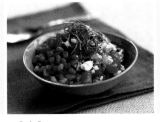
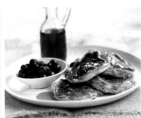

thursday	friday	saturday	sunday
1 slice low-calorie wholegrain toast with 2 tbsp low-sugar jam; 240ml (8fl oz) skimmed milk	60g (2½oz) low-sugar wholegrain cereal with 240ml (8fl oz) skimmed milk; 1 peach; 125ml (4fl oz) orange juice	2-egg vegetable omelette; 1 slice low-calorie wholemeal toast; 2 soya or vegetarian sausages; 125ml (4 fl oz) vegetable juice	2 Blueberry buckwheat pancakes (*see pp82–83*) with 2 tbsp maple syrup; 125ml (4fl oz) orange juice
1 slice low-calorie wholegrain toast with 2 tbsp low-fat cottage cheese or low-fat ricotta cheese	1 hard-boiled egg; 6 wholegrain crackers; 1 tbsp low-fat mayonnaise	30g (1oz) mozzarella cheese; 2 kiwi fruit	2 oatcakes with 1 tbsp peanut butter; ½ banana
1 serving Chicken and amaranth salad with tarragon and almonds (*see p94*); 6 wholegrain crackers	1 serving Artichoke, buckwheat noodle, and tofu salad (*see p95*)	115g (4oz) turkey breast burger in wholegrain wrap with mustard and sliced tomatoes	1 serving Toasted sweetcorn and bulgur salad with cherry tomatoes (*see p98*); 1 slice Soft rye bread (*see p143*)
125g (4½oz) wholewheat pasta with a tomato, capers, and mushroom sauce; garden salad with 2 tbsp low-fat dressing	170g (6oz) grilled chicken breast; 1 serving Barley risotto with vine-ripened tomatoes and feta (*see p130*); steamed courgettes	115g (4oz) filet mignon; 2 Oatcakes with goat's cheese and prunes (*see p107*); sliced tomatoes and avocado; steamed broccoli	170g (6oz) grilled tuna; 1 serving Garlic-ginger kale with quinoa and sesame (*see p137*); steamed peas and carrots
2 Oatmeal raisin cookies (*see pp150–51*)	1 nectarine	1 sliced peach with 100g (3½oz) low-fat yoghurt	2 handfuls air-popped popcorn

week 2

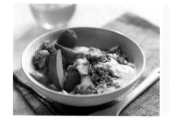 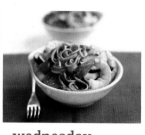

	monday	tuesday	wednesday
breakfast	1 serving Cinnamon-oat muesli with yoghurt, peaches, and raspberries (*see pp86–87*); 125ml (4fl oz) orange juice	1 Buckwheat crêpe with ham and low-fat cheese (*see p81*); ½ grapefruit; 240ml (8fl oz) skimmed milk	3 scrambled egg whites; 1 slice low-calorie wholemeal toast with 1 tsp low-fat margarine; 125ml (4fl oz) orange juice
snack	2 oatcakes with 1 tbsp low-sugar jam; ½ banana	1 wholegrain cereal bar; 240ml (8fl oz) skimmed milk	1 apple; 6 wholegrain crackers
lunch	1 serving Baby spinach, quinoa, and toasted pine nut salad (*see pp100–101*); 6 wholegrain crackers	2 Amaranth-courgette patties (*see p106*); 1 serving Hearty millet and butternut squash soup (*see pp92–93*)	3 Middle-Eastern meatballs with tomato sauce (*see pp124–25*); carrot and celery sticks with 2 tbsp low-fat dressing
dinner	1 serving Veal stew with millet, baby carrots, and thyme (*see pp128–29*); cucumber salad with 2 tbsp low-fat dressing	170g (6oz) grilled chicken with 1 serving Sweet pepper, sorghum, and pine nut pilaf (*see p136*); steamed string beans	1 serving Prawn soba primavera (*see pp118–19*); salad with 2 tbsp low-fat dressing
dessert or snack	30g (1oz) mozzarella cheese; 4 wholegrain crackers	200g (7oz) low-fat yoghurt with 125g (4½oz) fresh berries	2 handfuls air-popped popcorn

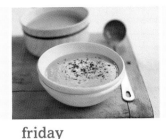

thursday	friday	saturday	sunday
60g (2¼oz) wholegrain cereal with 240ml (8fl oz) skimmed milk; ½ banana	225g (8oz) oatmeal porridge made with skimmed milk; 2 tbsp raisins; 125ml (4fl oz) orange juice	2 slices Wholegrain French toast with mango-kiwi fruit salsa (*see p90*) with 2 tbsp maple syrup; 240ml (8fl oz) skimmed milk	1 scrambled egg; 1 serving Sweetcorn and red potato breakfast fry (*see p84*); 125ml (4fl oz) vegetable juice
6 wholegrain crackers with 125g (4½oz) low-fat cottage cheese or low-fat ricotta cheese	2 plums; 200g (7oz) low-fat yoghurt	2 clementines	200g (7oz) low-fat yoghurt; 35g (1¼oz) raisins
1 serving Roasted aubergine and triticale salad with peanuts (*see p99*); 1 slice Nutty millet banana bread (*see pp144–45*)	1 serving Peppers stuffed with quinoa and minced turkey (*see p115*); tomato and cucumber salad with 2 tbsp low-fat dressing	1 Quinoa tuna salad sandwich on low-calorie wholemeal bread (*see p111*) with lettuce, tomato, and sprouts	1 serving Grecian spelt, cucumber, dill, and mint salad (*see pp102–103*); large garden salad with 2 tbsp low-fat dressing
1 slice Sweet tomato-glazed veggie loaf (*see p123*); tomato, avocado, onion, and basil salad; steamed broccoli	170g (6oz) grilled tuna; 1 serving Hearty millet and butternut squash soup (*see pp92–93*); 6 wholegrain crackers	170g (6oz) pork loin; 1 serving Lemon bulgur salad with chickpeas and roasted peppers (*see pp104–105*); salad with 2 tbsp low-fat dressing	1 serving Moroccan amaranth chicken stew (*see pp120–21*); 1 serving Pepper, courgette, and buckwheat sauté (*see pp138–39*)
140g (5oz) strawberries (fresh or frozen)	2 plums	1 slice Nutty millet banana bread (*see pp144–45*)	1 slice Pear hazelnut crisp (*see pp152–53*); 2 tbsp low-fat vanilla frozen yoghurt

week 3

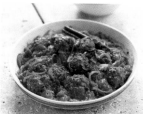

	monday	tuesday	wednesday
breakfast	60g (2¼oz) low-sugar, wholegrain cereal with 240ml (8fl oz) skimmed milk; 1 small sliced banana	1 serving Cinnamon-oat muesli with yoghurt, peaches, and raspberries (*see p86–87*); 125ml (4fl oz) orange juice	225g (8oz) oatmeal porridge made with skimmed milk with 2 tbsp raisins and 1 tbsp maple syrup; 125ml (4oz) orange juice
snack	2 oatcakes with 1 tbsp peanut butter; 1 orange	2 wholegrain cookies	225g (8oz) fresh fruit salad
lunch	3 Middle-Eastern meatballs (*see pp124–5*) with 125g (4½oz) wholewheat pasta and tomato sauce; salad with 2 tbsp low-fat dressing	1 serving Courgette, barley, and mushroom soup (*see p91*); 6 wholegrain crackers	2 Amaranth-courgette patties (*see p106*); 1 serving Hearty millet and butternut squash soup (*see pp92–93*)
dinner	170g (6oz) grilled salmon, 1 serving Barley with leeks and fennel (*see pp 132–33*); steamed asparagus	1 serving Moroccan amaranth chicken stew (*see pp120–21*); sliced tomato, onion, and avocado salad; steamed peas and carrots	1 slice Sweet tomato-glazed veggie loaf (*see pp123*); 1 serving Baby spinach, quinoa, and toasted pine nut salad (*see pp100–101*)
dessert or snack	2 scoops sorbet	2 sliced peaches with 100g (3½oz) natural yoghurt	1 slice Nutty millet banana bread (*see pp144–45*)

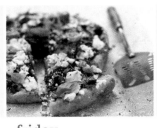 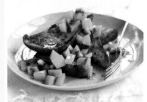

thursday	friday	saturday	sunday
1 Banana-walnut oatbran muffin (*see pp88–89*); 1 hard-boiled egg; 240ml (8fl oz) skimmed milk	60g (2½oz) low-sugar, wholegrain cereal with 240ml (8fl oz) skimmed milk; 1 peach	1 serving Wholegrain corn huevos rancheros (*see p85*); ½ serving Sweetcorn and red potato breakfast fry (*see p84*); ½ grapefruit; 240ml (8fl oz) skimmed milk	2 slices Wholegrain French toast with mango-kiwi fruit salsa (*p90*) with 2 tbsp maple syrup; 240ml (8fl oz) skimmed milk
200g (7oz) low-fat yoghurt with 125g (4½oz) fresh berries	1 small banana; 35g (1¼oz) unsalted almonds	1 hard-boiled egg; 6 wholegrain crackers; 1 tbsp low-fat mayonnaise	2 clementines
1 serving Sweetcorn, barley, and rocket salad with goat's cheese (*see pp96–97)*; steamed cauliflower	1 Quinoa tuna salad sandwich on low-calorie wholemeal bread (*see p111*) with 1 tbsp low-fat mayonnaise	2 Polenta crusted oven-fried chicken fingers (*see pp 112–13*); 1 slice Southwestern-style American cornbread (*see p142*); steamed Swiss chard	1 serving Toasted sweetcorn and bulgur salad with cherry tomatoes (*see p98*); 1 slice Soft rye bread (*see p143*)
1 serving Prawn soba primavera (*see pp118–19*); salad with 2 tbsp low-fat dressing	1 slice Spinach and goat's cheese wholegrain pizza (*see pp126–27*); salad with 2 tbsp low-fat dressing	170g (6oz) grilled chicken breast; 1 serving Barley risotto with vine-ripened tomatoes and feta (*see p130*); steamed peas	1 serving Italian-inspired barley with escarole and turkey sausage (*see p114*); salad with 2 tbsp low-fat dressing
1 handful air-popped popcorn	1 sliced cantaloupe melon	3 kiwi fruit	1 sliced apple topped with 100g (3½oz) low-fat yoghurt and muesli

week 4

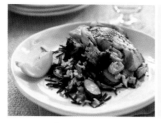 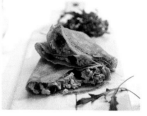

	monday	tuesday	wednesday
breakfast	1 serving Cinnamon-oat muesli with yoghurt, peaches, and raspberries (*see pp86–87*)	1 slice Southwestern-style American cornbread (*see p142*); 1 hard-boiled egg; 240ml (8fl oz) skimmed milk	1 slice nutty millet banana bread (*see pp144–45*) with 1 tbsp peanut butter; 240ml (8fl oz) skimmed milk
snack	60g (2½oz) low-sugar wholegrain cereal with 240ml (8fl oz) skimmed milk	200g (7oz) low-fat yoghurt with 60g (2¼oz) fresh berries	30g (1oz) mozzarella cheese; ½ grapefruit
lunch	1 serving Courgette, barley, and mushroom soup (*see p91*); 2 Amaranth-courgette patties (*see p106*)	1 Quinoa tuna salad sandwich on low-calorie wholemeal bread (*see p111*) with lettuce, tomato, and sprouts	2 Buckwheat crêpes with goat's cheese and sun-dried tomatoes (*see p110*); 200g (7oz) low-fat yoghurt
dinner	Sesame brown and wild rice with salmon (*see pp116–17*); steamed red and green peppers	1 serving Moroccan amaranth chicken stew (*see pp120–21*); 1 serving Citrus-pistachio spelt pilaf (*see pp134–35*); steamed spinach	115g (4oz) grilled sirloin steak; 1 serving Millet mashers (*see p131*); steamed fennel and cauliflower
dessert or snack	1 orange	2 Oatmeal raisin cookies (*see pp150–51*)	125g (4½oz) fresh berries with 2 tbsp low-fat vanilla frozen yoghurt

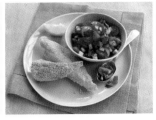

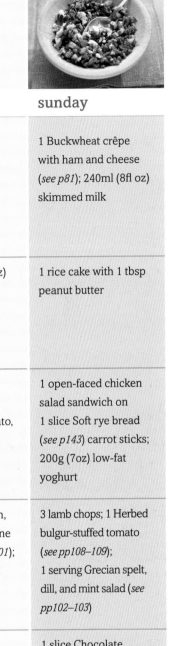

thursday	friday	saturday	sunday
1 slice Wholegrain French toast with mango-kiwi fruit salsa (*see p90*) with 1 tbsp maple syrup; 240ml (8fl oz) skimmed milk	1 scrambled egg; 1 serving Sweetcorn and red potato breakfast fry (*see p84*); 125ml (4fl oz) vegetable juice	1 serving Savoury amaranth porridge (*see p80*); 2 scrambled egg whites with tomatoes; 125ml (4fl oz) orange juice	1 Buckwheat crêpe with ham and cheese (*see p81*); 240ml (8fl oz) skimmed milk
3 kiwi fruit	2 tbsp unsalted almonds; 200g (7oz) low-fat yoghurt	1 banana; 240ml (8fl oz) skimmed milk	1 rice cake with 1 tbsp peanut butter
115g (4oz) grilled chicken breast; 1 serving Barley with leeks and fennel (*see pp132–33*)	2 Polenta-crusted oven-fried chicken fingers (*see pp112–13*); 1 slice Southwestern-style American cornbread (*see p142*)	1 slice Sweet tomato-glazed veggie loaf (*see p123*); cucumber, tomato, and basil salad	1 open-faced chicken salad sandwich on 1 slice Soft rye bread (*see p143*) carrot sticks; 200g (7oz) low-fat yoghurt
1 serving Peppers stuffed with quinoa and minced turkey (*see p115*); salad with 2 tbsp low-fat dressing; steamed mangetout	170g (6oz) grilled tuna; 1 serving Curried squash risotto with brown and wild rice (*see pp140–41*); steamed string beans	1 serving Baby spinach, quinoa, and toasted pine nut salad (*see pp100–101*); 2 Oatcakes with goat's cheese and prunes (*see p107*)	3 lamb chops; 1 Herbed bulgur-stuffed tomato (*see pp108–109*); 1 serving Grecian spelt, dill, and mint salad (*see pp102–103*)
1 mango with 200g (7oz) low-fat yoghurt	2 thick slices fresh watermelon	1 apple; 200g (7oz) low-fat yoghurt	1 slice Chocolate peanut butter pie (*see p149*)

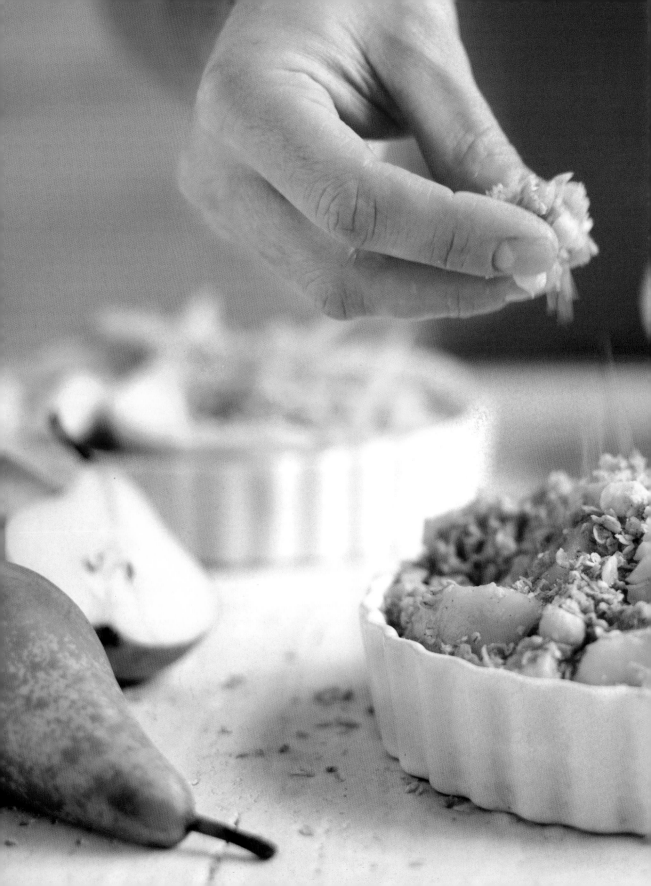

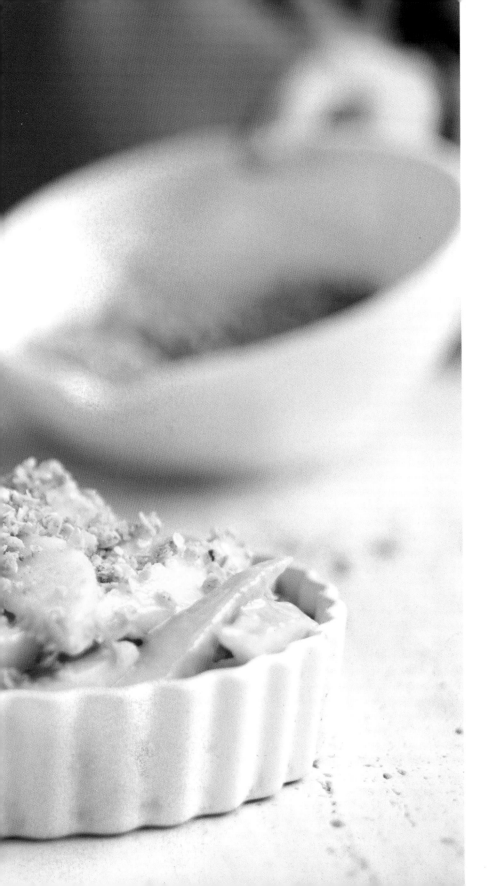

the recipes

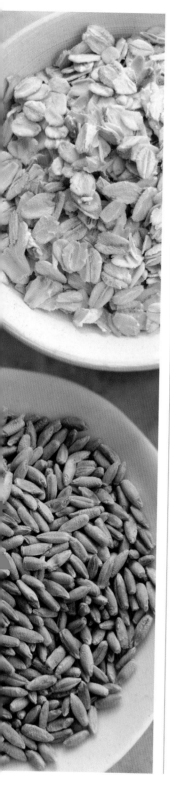

buying, storing, and baking with wholegrains

Most dried wholegrains have a very long shelf-life, so feel free to stock up on bags of wholegrains from your local health food shop. And if you can't find the kind of wholegrain flour you require, try grinding your own from the wholegrains themselves, using the directions below.

Identifying and buying wholegrains

The packaging and marketing terminology on pre-prepared food labels can be tricky to de-code so, whenever possible, buy raw wholegrains in their least processed form. Look for the word "whole" in front of the type of grain in the ingredients list, such as "whole barley" or "whole oats", and ideally this should be the first ingredient listed. Phrases such as "100 per cent rye" typically mean that rye is the only grain in the product, but it doesn't mean that the rye is wholegrain. Similarly, a product labelled "multigrain", "bran", or "pumpernickel" may not necessarily contain wholegrains as it may just contain different refined grains mixed together.

The term "stoneground", which is a technique for grinding grains, does not ensure that the grain remains whole, as sometimes the bran is removed first. Do not trust a food's colour, either, to determine whether it is made from wholegrains as the dark colour may result from artificial food colourings or molasses. (And some wholegrains, such as oats and amaranth, are naturally light in colour.) To ensure that your food contains wholegrain flour, you can always make your own. Simply place your wholegrains in a coffee grinder and grind until you achieve a fine, flour-like powder.

Storing wholegrains and flours

Most wholegrains, if stored uncooked in an airtight container in the refrigerator, can last for up to six months, and some, such as barley, can last up to a year. Some wholegrains, such as barley, quinoa, and brown rice, can be stored in an airtight container in a cool, dry place and will remain fresh for 6–12 months. However, if you live in a hot, humid climate, always store wholegrain products in the refrigerator or freezer.

Buckwheat flour should be stored in the refrigerator and will keep fresh for several months. Millet and oat flours may turn rancid quickly, so it is recommended to buy the grains and grind them right before use, rather than storing for long periods. It is best not to let corn sit around for too long after buying it as it tends to lose its flavour quickly – cook and serve it as soon as possible. Refrigerate the corn in plastic bags and don't remove the husks until just before cooking. It is possible to freeze ears of corn for up to one year. Simply blanch them in boiling water for eight minutes, then place them in sturdy freezer bags before freezing. To store popcorn, keep the kernels out of direct sunlight in an airtight container, as they can lose the moisture that allows them to pop so well.

Baking with gluten-free flours

If you want to avoid gluten, there is a range of wholegrain gluten-free flours to choose from. Whole cornmeal produces moist and delicious breads, muffins, and biscuits, and buckwheat flour, with its delicate nutty flavour, is ideal for use in pancakes, pie crusts, breads, and brownies.

Amaranth flour does not lose nutrients when processed and teff flour is light in flavour and texture. Flours made from millet or sorghum enrich baked goods with vitamins and minerals without changing the flavour. Brown rice flour is great for baking delicate breads and pizza crusts, while quinoa flour imparts a lovely moistness to baked goods.

Bear in mind that gluten-free flours work best in recipes for non-yeast breads, such as pancakes and flatbreads. This is because gluten gives baked goods elasticity, which allows them to rise without breaking. If you need to make gluten-free breads rise, you can add xanthan gum or guar gum to the recipe.

Baking with flours that contain gluten

Wholegrain flours that contain gluten can be used in a wide variety of cooking and baking recipes, including yeast breads. To boost the nutrient content of your baked goods, simply replace half the amount of plain flour with wholegrain flour. If you wish, you can substitute the entire amount of plain flour with a wholegrain variety, but it may result in baked goods with lower volume and coarser texture.

Wholewheat and spelt flours are the most versatile wholegrain flours available, offering a variety of nutrients along with delicious flavour. Barley flour is sweet and nutty, while kamut flour has a rich, buttery flavour. Dark rye flour makes lovely, dense rye breads. Use triticale flour to make yeast breads, but make sure to cut the kneading time in half so as to not disrupt the delicate fermentation process. (Most triticale breads also require 5–10 minutes extra baking time.) Oat flour is delicious in cookies, pancakes, and muffins. Although oats do not contain gluten, they are typically grown in wheat fields, and are not recommended for people who are allergic to gluten.

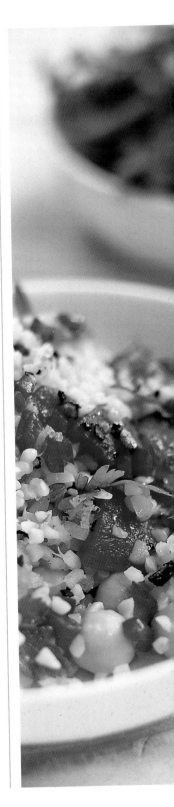

savoury amaranth porridge

serves 6

ingredients

750ml (1¼pts) reduced-sodium chicken stock

175ml (6fl oz) fat-free single cream

1 tbsp unsalted butter or margarine

195g (6¾oz) amaranth

⅛ tsp fine sea salt, or to taste

⅛ tsp freshly ground white pepper, or to taste

2 tbsp finely snipped fresh chives (optional)

alternative grains

Wholegrain cornmeal (polenta) can be used to prepare this dish. If you wish to add cheese to your dish, sprinkle a little low-fat grated Cheddar for the best taste.

Sprinkled with a little low-fat cheese, eaten as a side dish with eggs, or even made sweet with a light dusting of brown sugar, this creamy hot cereal provides a warming, filling start to the day. This is a great way to try amaranth for the first time.

1 **Bring the stock,** cream, and butter or margarine to the boil, then simmer in a medium-sized saucepan over a medium heat.

2 **Whisk in the amaranth.** Reduce the heat to low, cover, and cook for 25 minutes. Remove the lid and cook for an additional 10 minutes, stirring occasionally, or until it reaches the desired consistency. Remove from the heat and leave to stand for five minutes.

3 **Add salt and pepper** to taste. If using, stir in the chives and serve while hot.

nutritional analysis per serving: calories 170; calories from fat 35; total fat 4g; saturated fat 1g; cholesterol 0mg; sodium 360mg; carbohydrates 24g; dietary fibre 5g; protein 7g.

buckwheat crêpes with ham and cheese

serves 6
makes 6 crêpes

ingredients

1 large egg

150ml (5fl oz) cold skimmed milk

1 tbsp unsalted butter or margarine, melted

35g (1¼oz) buckwheat flour

35g (1¼oz) unbleached plain flour

1 tbsp rapeseed oil

1 tbsp Dijon mustard, or to taste

6 slices natural, lean, baked ham or turkey ham, halved

115g (4oz) grated Gruyère or other Swiss cheese

½ tsp freshly ground black pepper

alternative grains

For a darker, earthier crêpe, see Alternative grains on page 82. Another tasty option is to use wholewheat tortillas: fill each tortilla, then brush the tortillas with oil; cook in the oven or in a frying pan until the cheese melts.

There's nothing quite like the taste of freshly prepared crêpes. Consider it Parisian pleasure on a plate, one that is high in protein and a good source of calcium, selenium, and zinc. This dish is perfect for those lazy Sunday mornings.

1 **Blend the egg,** milk, butter or margarine, and flours at high speed for one minute, or until no lumps remain. Refrigerate, covered, for at least 1 hour.

2 **Add half a teaspoon of oil** to a non-stick crêpe pan or non-stick frying pan over a medium heat. Spoon about 3 tablespoons of batter into the pan, tilting the pan to coat. Cook for 1 minute or until the edges begin to pull away from the pan and the bottom is lightly browned. Flip the crêpe over and cook for 30 seconds, or until lightly browned. Repeat with the remaining oil and batter to make 6 crêpes. Preheat the oven to 180°C (350°F, gas 4).

3 **On top of each crêpe,** brush some Dijon mustard, add 2 halves of ham slices, and sprinkle with the cheese and pepper. Fold the edges over, place on a large tray and heat in the oven for 5 minutes, or until the cheese is melted. Serve warm.

nutritional analysis (1 crêpe): calories 200; calories from fat 110; total fat 12g; saturated fat 4.5g; cholesterol 75mg; sodium 410mg; carbohydrates 8g; dietary fibre 1g; protein 14g.

blueberry buckwheat pancakes

serves 3
makes 6 pancakes

ingredients

35g (1¼oz) buckwheat flour (plus 1 tbsp for tossing blueberries)

35g (1¼oz) unbleached plain flour

1 tsp double-acting baking powder

1 tbsp cold, unsalted butter, cut into pieces

1 tbsp acacia or orange blossom honey

1 large egg

90ml (3fl oz) vanilla-flavoured soya milk

115g (4oz) fresh, or frozen and thawed, blueberries (can also use diced green apples instead)

Oil cooking spray

2 tbsp maple syrup, warm (optional)

alternative grains

For a darker, earthier pancake, use 70g (2½oz) buckwheat flour instead of 35g (1¼oz) buckwheat flour plus 35g (1¼oz) plain flour.

The sweetness from the blueberries is a perfect complement to the nuttiness from the buckwheat flour. Enjoy these pancakes when fresh blueberries are at their peak or all year round with frozen berries, for lots of antioxidants and fibre.

1 **In a medium-sized bowl,** combine 35g (1¼oz) buckwheat flour, the plain flour, baking powder, butter, and honey into a fine crumbled mixture with a pastry blender or potato masher.

2 **In a large bowl,** whisk together the egg and soya milk. Add the flour mixture to the egg-soya milk mixture and whisk until the batter is well combined. Leave to stand for 5 minutes. Toss the blueberries with 1 tablespoon of buckwheat flour and stir into the batter.

3 **Preheat the oven** to 110°C (225°F, gas ¼). Coat a large, flat, non-stick frying pan or griddle with oil cooking spray. Place over a medium heat.

4 **Spoon the batter,** about 3 tablespoons per pancake, onto the hot surface. Cook the pancakes in batches, 2 minutes per side, or until cooked through. Transfer the cooked pancakes to a heatproof platter and keep warm in the oven. Serve with maple syrup, if desired.

nutritional analysis (2 pancakes): calories 190; calories from fat 60; total fat 6g; saturated fat 3g; cholesterol 80mg; sodium 220mg; carbohydrates 28g; dietary fibre 3g; protein 6g.

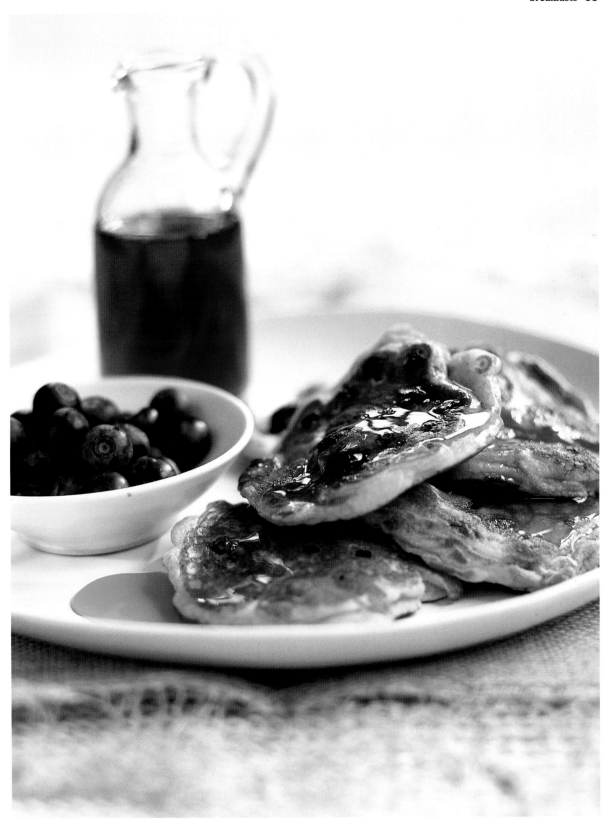

sweetcorn and red potato breakfast fry

serves 4

ingredients

1½ tbsp extra-virgin olive oil

1 small or ½ large red onion, finely chopped

1 small jalapeño pepper (remove half or all the seeds), finely chopped

2 large boiled red-skinned potatoes such as Desirée with skin, chilled and diced

125g (4½oz) frozen and thawed, or tinned, yellow sweetcorn, drained

½ tsp garlic salt, or to taste

15g (½oz) chopped fresh flat-leaf parsley

alternative grains

When fresh sweetcorn is plentiful, use fresh boiled sweetcorn in this recipe in place of tinned or frozen varieties.

This delicious recipe is a great way to increase your vegetable intake in the morning, or any time of the day. Based on traditional American hash browns, this is a much healthier variation, containing a lot less fat and more fibre, vitamins C, B₆, and K, and potassium.

1 **Add the oil** to a large non-stick frying pan over a medium-high heat. Once the oil is hot, add the onion and jalapeño pepper and sauté for 5 minutes, or until lightly browned.

2 **Add the potatoes** and sweetcorn and cook for 5 minutes, or until the potatoes are lightly browned, stirring the potato mixture occasionally.

3 **Add garlic salt** to taste and sprinkle with parsley.

nutritional analysis per serving: calories 210; calories from fat 50; total fat 6g; saturated fat 1g; cholesterol 0mg; sodium 135mg; carbohydrates 36g; dietary fibre 4g; protein 4g.

wholegrain corn huevos rancheros with salsa verde

**serves 4
makes 4 topped
tortillas**

ingredients

4 x 15cm (6in) diameter
wholegrain corn tortillas

Oil cooking spray

2 large eggs

3 large egg whites

¼ tsp freshly ground
black pepper, or to taste

1 tsp corn or extra-virgin
olive oil

55g (2oz) grated low-fat
Gouda cheese

½ Hass avocado, peeled,
diced

125ml (4fl oz) jar salsa
verde or tomato-based
salsa

2 tbsp chopped fresh
coriander

alternative grains

Use yellow or white
corn tortillas, or try
wholewheat tortillas,
too. Both are delicious
for this meal, as well as
for sandwiches and other
Mexican-inspired dishes
such as quesadillas.

*Corn tortillas are one of the most mouthwatering ways to eat corn.
So, go ahead, kickstart the day with this Mexican classic. These
huevos rancheros or "ranch eggs" are simple to make, a good
source of protein, and will leave you feeling satisfied for hours.*

1 **Preheat the oven** to 230°C (450°F, gas 8). For crisp tortillas, coat the
top and bottom of each tortilla with oil cooking spray. Place on a large
baking sheet and bake for 8 minutes (4 minutes per side), or until crisp
and lightly browned. Alternatively, for soft tortillas, warm them according
to the packet instructions.

2 **Meanwhile,** place a non-stick frying pan over a medium heat. In a
bowl, whisk together the eggs, egg whites, and pepper. Add oil to the
frying pan. Once hot, pour the eggs into the frying pan and scramble
until fully cooked.

3 **Place 1 portion** of eggs on top of each tortilla. Immediately, top
each with cheese, avocado, salsa, and coriander.

nutritional analysis (1 tortilla): calories 230; calories from fat 100; total fat 11g;
saturated fat 3.5g; cholesterol 115mg; sodium 380mg; carbohydrates 26g; dietary
fibre 4g; protein 14g.

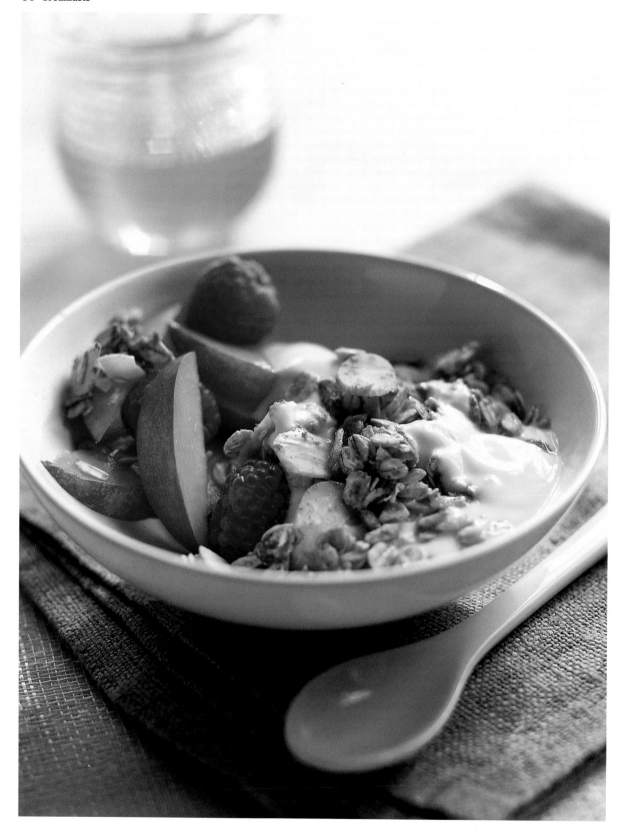

cinnamon-oat muesli with yoghurt, peaches, and raspberries

serves 4

ingredients

85g (3oz) rolled oats

30g (1oz) flaked almonds

2 tbsp wheat germ

2 tbsp shelled sunflower seeds, unsalted

1½ tsp ground cinnamon

3 tbsp acacia or orange blossom honey

250g (9oz) fresh, or frozen and thawed, diced peaches

475ml (16fl oz) fat-free and sugar-free peach or vanilla yoghurt

250g (9oz) fresh, or frozen and thawed, raspberries

alternative grains

Add an extra 25g (scant 1oz) oats if you don't want to use the wheat germ. Use other fresh or frozen fruits, such as blueberries or strawberries.

Indulge yourself with a morning treat for the taste buds. It's a balanced meal all in one that's bursting with wholesomeness from the protein, calcium, magnesium, iron, and zinc. A dish so tasty, you won't want to limit it to breakfast-time, since it also makes a great snack or dessert.

1 **Preheat the oven** to 160°C (325°F, gas 3).

2 **Thoroughly mix** the oats, almonds, wheat germ, sunflower seeds, and cinnamon in a medium-sized bowl. Continue to stir while drizzling the honey into the mixture until well combined.

3 **Spread the muesli mixture** evenly onto a non-stick 22x32cm (9x13in) baking tin. Bake for 25 minutes, or until golden brown, stirring occasionally during baking. Remove from the oven and leave to cool slightly. (Makes 280g/10oz muesli.)

4 **Arrange the peaches** in bowls and top with the yoghurt, muesli, and raspberries. Experiment with various fruits and yoghurts, if desired.

nutritional analysis per serving: calories 280; calories from fat 60g; total fat 7g; saturated fat 0.5g; cholesterol 0mg; sodium 65mg; carbohydrates 47g; dietary fibre 5g; protein 10g.

banana-walnut oat bran muffins

serves 12
makes 12 muffins

ingredients

4 tbsp corn or
rapeseed oil

200g (7oz) granulated
sugar

2 large eggs, well beaten

85g (3oz) rolled oats

140g (5oz) unbleached
plain flour

25g (scant 1oz) oat bran

1 tsp bicarbonate of soda

¼ tsp fine sea salt

3 large fully ripened
bananas, peeled and
mashed

2 tsp pure vanilla extract

Oil cooking spray

45g (1½oz) chopped
walnuts

alternative grains

Instead of 140g (5oz)
unbleached plain flour,
use 90g (3¾oz)
unbleached plain
flour plus 35g (1¼oz)
wholemeal flour. Also,
in place of oat bran, try
wholegrain cornmeal
(polenta).

These perfectly portioned muffins are light on fat, but heavy on flavour. The vitamins and minerals from the oats will give you energy, and the fibre will keep your stomach feeling full and satisfied, providing you with an excellent start to the day.

1 **Preheat the oven** to 180°C (350°F, gas 4). In a large mixing bowl, blend together the oil and sugar. Add the beaten eggs and blend well.

2 **In a separate bowl,** mix together the oats, flour, oat bran, bicarbonate of soda, and salt. Add the dry ingredients to the egg mixture and mix with a large spoon until combined. Add the bananas and vanilla extract and stir until just combined.

3 **Lightly coat** a 12-hole non-stick muffin tin or deep bun tray with oil cooking spray. Spoon the mixture into the prepared tin, filling the individual compartments to one-quarter full. Press the walnuts on top of the muffin mixture.

4 **Bake the muffins** in the middle of the oven for 25 minutes, or until the tops are golden and the tester comes out clean. Cool the muffins in the tin on a rack for 10 minutes. Remove the muffins from the tin and leave to cool on the rack.

nutritional analysis (1 muffin): calories 220; calories from fat 70; total fat 8g; saturated fat 1g; cholesterol 35mg; sodium 170mg; carbohydrates 36g; dietary fibre 2g; protein 4g.

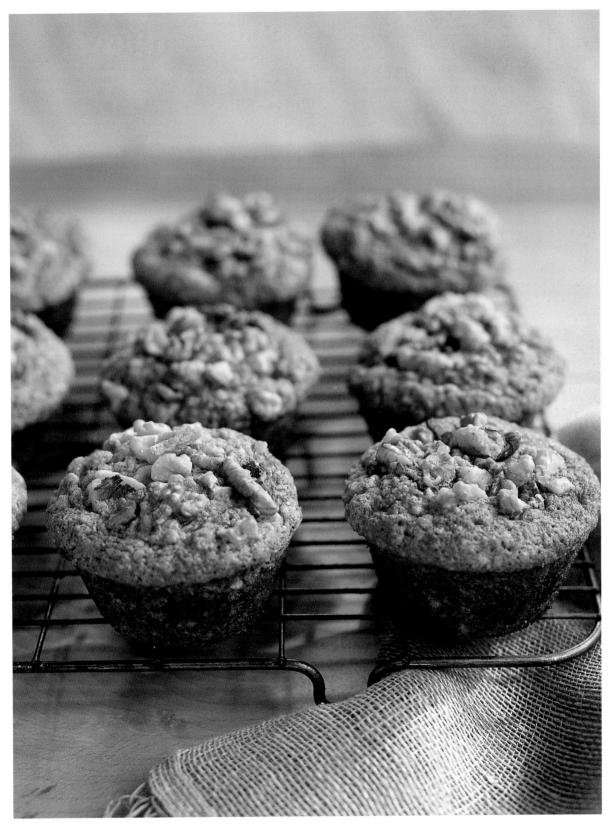

wholegrain french toast with mango-kiwi fruit salsa

serves 4

ingredients

2 large eggs

4 large egg whites

90ml (3fl oz) vanilla-flavoured soya milk

90ml (3fl oz) apricot nectar or 60ml (2fl oz) fresh orange juice mixed with 2 tbsp apricot jam

8 slices granary, low-calorie bread

1 medium mango, peeled and diced

2 medium kiwi fruit, peeled and diced

1 tbsp pure maple syrup, or to taste

4 tsp unsalted butter

alternative grains

Try with various types of wholegrain breads, including wholemeal and oatmeal bread. To reduce calories, use sugar-free or "light" maple syrup, and use oil spray cooking instead of butter in the pan.

Perhaps a better name for this breakfast is Tropical Toast. The mango and kiwi fruit provide 100 per cent of the recommended vitamin C requirements for one day. This breakfast is also rich in B vitamins, the minerals selenium and manganese, as well as fibre.

1 **In a medium-sized bowl,** whisk the eggs, egg whites, soya milk, and apricot nectar or orange juice mixture. Arrange the bread in two 22x32cm (9x13in) baking tins. Evenly distribute the egg mixture over the bread, flipping the slices over to coat both sides. Cover with cling film and refrigerate for at least 30 minutes, or overnight.

2 **Meanwhile,** gently stir the mango, kiwi fruit, and maple syrup in a small bowl for the salsa; set aside.

3 **Melt 1 teaspoon of butter** in a large, flat, non-stick frying pan over a medium heat. Add the bread to the pan in batches and cook for 2 minutes per side, or until golden brown, adding more butter to the pan as necessary.

4 **Transfer** to a platter. Top each with about 3 tablespoons of salsa when serving. Drizzle with additional maple syrup, if desired.

nutritional analysis (2 slices): calories 270; calories from fat 70; total fat 8g; saturated fat 1.5g; cholesterol 110mg; sodium 340mg; carbohydrates 42g; dietary fibre 7g; protein 12g.

courgette, barley, and mushroom soup

serves 6

ingredients

2 tbsp extra-virgin
olive oil

1 large white onion, sliced

2 large garlic cloves,
finely chopped

1.8 litres (scant 3¼pts)
reduced-sodium beef
stock

1 bay leaf

200g (7oz) lightly
pearled barley

225g (8oz) fresh chestnut
mushrooms, thinly sliced

1 medium courgette,
cut lengthways and
thinly sliced

1 tsp chopped
fresh thyme

2 tbsp chopped fresh
parsley

alternative grains

Try this soup with the
wholegrain hulled barley.
However, note that it will
take significantly longer
to cook – about 1½ hours.
Additional stock will
likely be needed.

This pleasantly filling vegetable and barley-packed soup is healthiest and tastes best when courgettes are in season. It's also loaded with plenty of fibre, vitamins C and K, and minerals such as selenium, potassium, and manganese.

1 **Add the oil** to a stockpot or large saucepan over a medium heat. Once the oil is hot, add the onion and sauté for 5 minutes. Add the garlic and sauté for 1 minute.

2 **Add the stock,** 475ml (16fl oz) water, bay leaf, and barley and bring to the boil over a high heat. Reduce the heat to medium, cover, and cook for 50 minutes, or until the barley is nearly tender. Remove the bay leaf.

3 **Add the mushrooms,** courgette, and thyme and cook, covered, for 8 minutes, or until the vegetables and barley are tender. If necessary, add more stock until it is the desired consistency.

4 **Ladle the soup** into bowls. Sprinkle with parsley.

nutritional analysis per serving: calories 230; calories from fat 60; total fat 7g; saturated fat 1.5g; cholesterol 0mg; sodium 105mg; carbohydrates 32g; dietary fibre 6g; protein 11g.

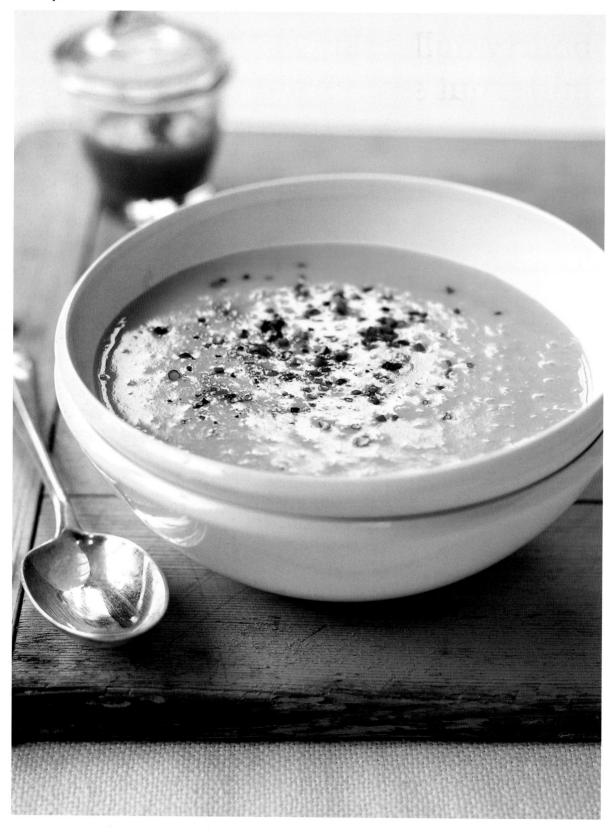

hearty millet and butternut squash soup

serves 8

ingredients

1.3 litres (2¼ pts) reduced-sodium chicken or vegetable stock

150g (5½oz) millet

1 medium butternut squash, peeled, seeded, and cut into cubes

240ml (8fl oz) low-fat plain soya milk

¼ tsp hot pepper sauce, or to taste

¼ tsp salt, or to taste

3 tbsp finely snipped fresh chives

alternative grains

This soup will be lovely with amaranth in place of millet – and creamier, too.

Millet is considered one of the oldest grains in the world. But this soup, with its brilliant orange colour and creamy yet millet-studded texture, is thoroughly modern. This soup supplies 400 per cent of your daily requirement for vitamin A, and 70 per cent of your vitamin C needs.

1 **In a large stockpot** or saucepan, bring the stock to the boil over a high heat. Add the millet and simmer, covered, over a medium-low heat for 30 minutes, or until the millet is well cooked.

2 **Add the squash** and soya milk and stir. Simmer, covered, for another 30 minutes, or until the squash is fork-tender.

3 **Purée the mixture** in the pot using a hand-held blender. Alternatively, purée the slightly cooled soup mixture in batches in a freestanding blender or food processor until creamy. Then transfer the puréed soup into a separate stockpot or saucepan.

4 **If necessary,** add more stock until you achieve the desired consistency. To the simmering soup, add hot pepper sauce and salt to taste. Stir in or top with chives.

nutritional analysis per serving: calories 180; calories from fat 10; total fat 1g; saturated fat 0g; cholesterol 0mg; sodium 410mg; carbohydrates 39g; dietary fibre 6g; protein 7g.

chicken and amaranth salad with tarragon and almonds

serves 4

ingredients

60g (2¼oz) amaranth

340g (12oz) poached or roasted boneless, skinless chicken breast, cut into cubes, chilled

1 celery stick, thinly sliced

45g (1½oz) finely chopped onion

90ml (3fl oz) fat-free soured cream

2 tbsp reduced-fat mayonnaise

2 tbsp fat-free natural yoghurt

1 tbsp apple cider vinegar

1 tbsp chopped fresh tarragon, or to taste

Pinch of salt (optional)

4 large Little Gem or other lettuce leaves

25g (scant 1oz) flaked almonds, toasted

alternative grains

Quinoa or millet are both good alternatives to amaranth in this salad.

Amaranth is a lovely grain that provides a caviar-like texture, and it makes this chicken salad like no other. This salad is high in protein and a rich source of niacin, vitamin B₆, selenium, and magnesium. Try serving it with slices of toasted wholemeal bread.

1 **In a small saucepan** over a medium-high heat, bring the amaranth and 240ml (8fl oz) water to the boil; reduce the heat to medium-low and cover. Simmer for 15 minutes, or until tender. Remove from the heat and leave to stand for 5 minutes covered. Transfer to a bowl. Chill.

2 **In another bowl,** combine the chicken, celery, and onion.

3 **Mix the soured cream,** mayonnaise, yoghurt, vinegar, and tarragon into the amaranth. Combine with the chicken mixture. Refrigerate for at least 30 minutes before serving to allow the flavours to combine. Add salt to taste.

4 **Serve a portion** of the chicken and amaranth salad on each lettuce leaf. Sprinkle with almonds.

nutritional analysis per serving: calories 240; calories from fat 80; total fat 8g; saturated fat 1.5g; cholesterol 45mg; sodium 150mg; carbohydrates 19g; dietary fibre 4g; protein 22g.

artichoke, buckwheat noodle, and tofu salad

serves 6

ingredients

90ml (3fl oz) rice vinegar

2 tbsp finely chopped shallots

225g (8oz) dry buckwheat soba noodles

1½ tbsp extra-virgin olive oil

170g (6oz) thinly sliced, frozen and thawed, or tinned, water-packed artichoke hearts, drained

½ of 400g (14oz) packet (drained weight), firm tofu, drained and cut into cubes

20g (¾oz) finely sliced or chopped fresh basil, plus additional for garnish

3 tbsp pine nuts, toasted

⅛ tsp fine sea salt, or to taste

alternative grains

Enjoy with various types of pasta such as wholewheat linguine, fettucini, or udon noodles.

This zingy buckwheat soba noodle dish has everything you could ask for in a salad – flavour appeal, eye appeal, and nutritional appeal. It contains a good amount of protein as well as a range of minerals. Plus, the pine nuts provide texture and taste great.

1 **In a small bowl,** whisk the vinegar and shallots; set aside.

2 **Cook the noodles** in boiling water until al dente – approximately 1 minute less than suggested by the packet instructions. Drain. Toss the noodles in a large bowl with 1 tablespoon of oil. Toss with the vinegar-shallot mixture and artichoke hearts. Chill.

3 **Meanwhile,** in a non-stick frying pan over a medium heat, add the remaining oil. Once the oil is hot, add the tofu cubes. Sauté for 10 minutes, or until golden brown on all sides. Remove from the pan.

4 **Toss the noodles** with the tofu cubes, basil, and pine nuts. Add salt to taste. Serve chilled or at room temperature. Garnish with additional basil.

nutritional analysis per serving: calories 240; calories from fat 80; total fat 9g; saturated fat 1g; cholesterol 0mg; sodium 540mg; carbohydrates 33g; dietary fibre 2g; protein 11g.

sweetcorn, barley, and rocket salad with goat's cheese

serves 6

ingredients

100g (3½oz) lightly pearled barley

2 bunches rocket, coarsely chopped

170g (6oz) fresh sweetcorn (cooked, chilled, and cut from cob) or frozen and thawed, sweetcorn kernels

15g (½oz) snipped fresh chives

2 tbsp extra-virgin olive oil

3 tbsp apple cider vinegar

3 tbsp finely chopped shallots

2 tsp Dijon mustard

¼ tsp fine sea salt, or to taste

¼ tsp freshly ground black pepper, or to taste

85g (3oz) soft low-fat goat's cheese, crumbled

alternative grains

Spelt or triticale berries would provide a similar texture to this salad.

A perfect picnic or party food, this piquant salad tastes best (and is most nutritious) when made with fresh, in-season sweetcorn. The barley bumps up its fibre content, while fresh rocket gives it a zesty bite. For a real culinary treat, try making it with barbecued corn on the cob.

1 **In a medium-sized saucepan** over a high heat, bring the barley and about 500ml (17fl oz) water to the boil; reduce the heat to medium-low and cover. Simmer for 45 minutes, or until chewy yet tender. Remove from the heat and leave to stand for 10 minutes covered. Transfer to a bowl. Chill. (Note: this step can be done in advance.)

2 **In a large bowl,** mix the chilled barley with the rocket, corn, and chives.

3 **Whisk the oil,** vinegar, shallots, and mustard in a small bowl. Pour the dressing over the barley mixture to coat.

4 **Add salt and pepper.** Sprinkle with goat's cheese.

nutritional analysis per serving: calories 170; calories from fat 60; total fat 7g; saturated fat 2g; cholesterol 0mg; sodium 110mg; carbohydrates 23g; dietary fibre 5g; protein 5g.

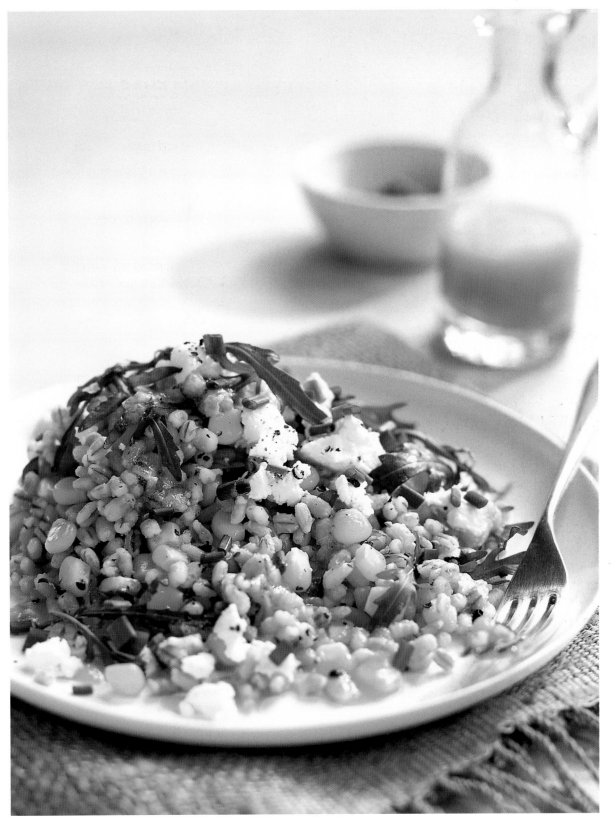

toasted sweetcorn and bulgur salad with cherry tomatoes

serves 4

ingredients

100g (3½oz) medium-grain bulgur

240ml (8fl oz) tomato juice

1 tbsp extra-virgin olive oil

125g (4½oz) fresh sweetcorn (cooked, chilled, and cut from cob) or frozen and thawed sweetcorn kernels

115g (4oz) cherry tomatoes, ½ very thinly sliced, ½ halved

15g (½oz) snipped fresh chives

15g (½oz) chopped or thinly sliced fresh basil

2 tbsp aged red wine vinegar, or to taste

1 tsp freshly ground black pepper, or to taste

alternative grains

Quinoa would work nicely in this salad. Or make sweetcorn the star. Skip the bulgur and tomato juice, use 325g (11½oz) sweetcorn, and keep everything else the same.

This salad is highly nutritious because of the vitamins A, C, and K, as well as magnesium and fibre. Toasting the bulgur in this salad adds nuttiness. Toasting the sweetcorn – also considered caramelizing – adds a natural sweetness.

1 **In a large frying pan,** toast the bulgur over a medium heat for 6 minutes, or until lightly browned, stirring occasionally.

2 **Add the tomato juice** and 125ml (4fl oz) water and bring to the boil. Reduce the heat and simmer, covered, for 5 minutes. Remove from the heat, keep covered, and leave to stand for 10 minutes to cool. Transfer to a bowl and chill.

3 **Add the oil** to a frying pan over a medium-high heat. Once the oil is hot, sauté the sweetcorn for 2 minutes, or until golden brown. Chill.

4 **Gently stir the sweetcorn,** very thinly sliced tomatoes, chives, basil, and vinegar into the bulgur. Add pepper to taste. Serve with halved tomatoes arranged on top of the salad.

nutritional analysis per serving: calories 160; calories from fat 35; total fat 4g; saturated fat 0.5g; cholesterol 0mg; sodium 170mg; carbohydrates 29g; dietary fibre 6g; protein 5g.

roasted aubergine and triticale salad with peanuts

serves 4

ingredients

25g (scant 1oz) triticale berries

4 Japanese aubergines

Juice of 1½ limes (about 3 tbsp)

3 tbsp thinly sliced shallots

2 spring onions, thinly sliced (green and white parts)

2 tbsp chopped fresh coriander, plus additional sprigs for garnish

1 tbsp garlic-chilli sauce

1 tbsp acacia or orange blossom honey

2 tsp natural, low-sodium soy sauce

2 tbsp chopped, unsalted, roasted nuts

alternative grains

Spelt is hearty enough to be showcased like triticale in this Japanese-inspired salad. Prepare it as you would the triticale.

Few people are familiar with triticale, and it is sometimes difficult to find, but this grain is an excellent source of fibre and contains lots of vitamins and minerals. If your local health food shop does not carry triticale, this salad would work equally well using spelt.

1 **In a small saucepan** over a high heat, bring the triticale and 475ml (16fl oz) water to the boil; reduce the heat to medium-low and cover. Simmer for 1 hour, or until chewy yet tender. Remove from the heat and leave to stand for 10 minutes covered. Transfer to a bowl. Chill.

2 **Preheat the oven** to 200°C (400°F, gas 6). Wrap each aubergine in foil and roast in the oven for 20 minutes, or until cooked through. Chill.

3 **Meanwhile,** place the lime juice, shallots, spring onions, coriander, garlic-chilli sauce, honey, and soy sauce in a medium-sized bowl and stir to combine. Cut off the stem of each chilled aubergine. Slice each aubergine in half lengthways; cut each half into 2 or 3 slices lengthways, then into small bite-sized pieces crossways. Toss the aubergine pieces and triticale with the mixture in the medium-sized bowl until coated.

4 **Before serving,** top with peanuts and garnish with coriander sprigs.

nutritional analysis per serving: calories 140; calories from fat 25; total fat 3g; saturated fat 0g; cholesterol 0mg; sodium 210mg; carbohydrates 27g; dietary fibre 7g; protein 5g.

baby spinach, quinoa, and toasted pine nut salad

serves 6

ingredients

140g (5oz) quinoa

Juice of 1 lemon (about 3 tbsp)

3 tbsp extra-virgin olive oil

⅛ tsp fine sea salt, or to taste

60g (2¼oz) fresh baby spinach

30g (1oz) feta cheese, crumbled

55g (2oz) finely sliced spring onions (about 3)

55g (2oz) cherry tomatoes, quartered

3 tbsp finely chopped fresh mint or basil (or mixture)

3 tbsp pine nuts, toasted

alternative grains

Bulgur or amaranth would work well in place of quinoa in this recipe.

As quinoa is considered by many to be the world's healthiest grain, this quinoa dish might be the world's healthiest salad. It's packed with vitamins, minerals, and protein. Serve this salad with Hearty millet and butternut squash soup (see pp92–93) for a tasty light meal.

1 **In a medium-sized saucepan,** over a high heat, bring the quinoa and 475ml (16fl oz) water to the boil; reduce the heat to medium and cover. Cook for 12 minutes, or until tender. Remove from the heat and leave to stand for 5 minutes covered.

2 **Meanwhile,** whisk the lemon juice, oil, and salt in a large bowl. Add the hot quinoa to the dressing and stir with a fork. Chill.

3 **Toss the chilled quinoa** with spinach, feta, spring onions, tomatoes, and herbs.

4 **Top with pine nuts** and serve.

nutritional analysis per serving: calories 230; calories from fat 120; total fat 13g; saturated fat 3g; cholesterol 5mg; sodium 160mg; carbohydrates 23g; dietary fibre 3g; protein 6g.

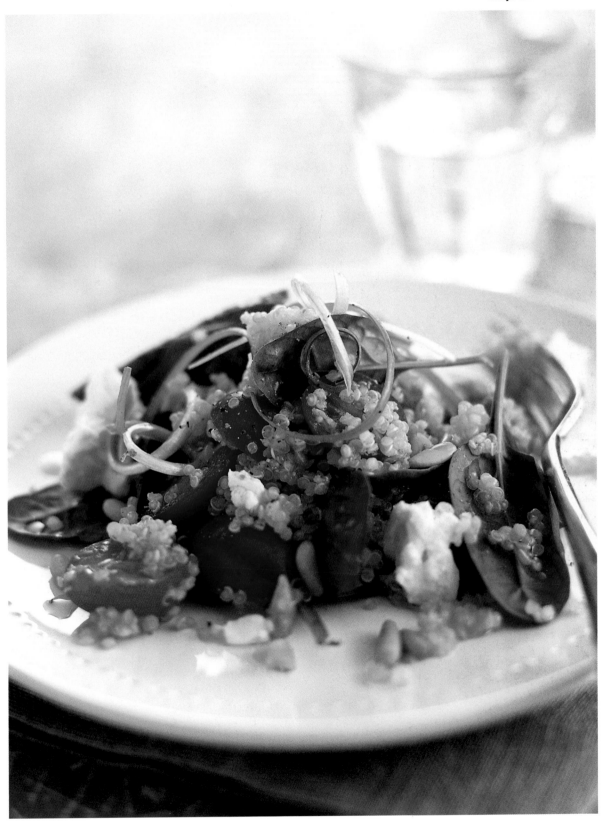

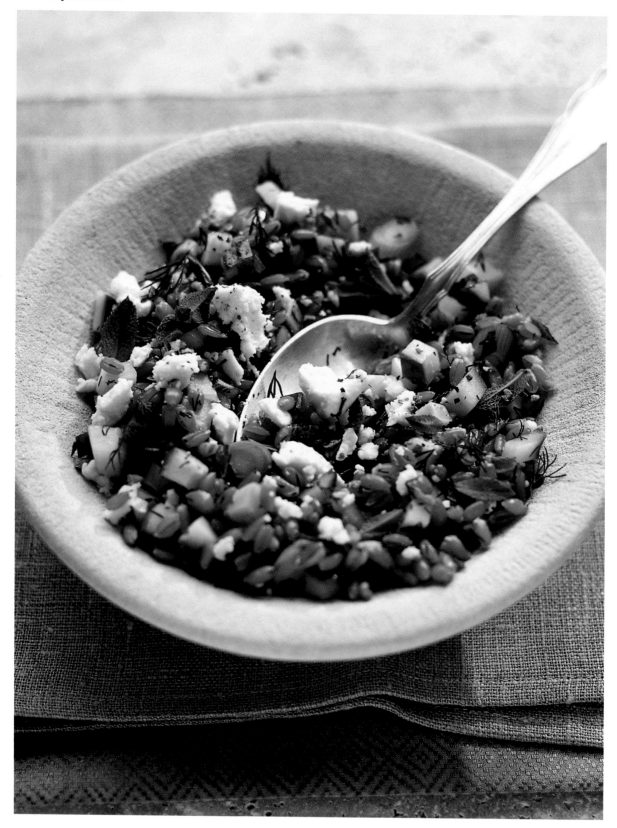

grecian spelt, cucumber, dill, and mint salad

serves 4

ingredients

45g (1½oz) spelt

4 tbsp fresh lemon juice

2 tbsp extra-virgin olive oil

1 large garlic clove, finely chopped

½ of 35cm (14in) cucumber, diced

55g (2oz) chopped spring onions (about 3)

15g (½oz) chopped fresh dill

15g (½oz) chopped fresh mint

½ tsp freshly ground black pepper, or to taste

¼ tsp fine sea salt, or to taste

25g (scant 1oz) crumbled feta cheese

alternative grain

Make this salad more like traditional tabbouleh by using bulgur. Try triticale for a bigger bite, or even brown rice.

This Greek twist on a tabbouleh salad is made with crumbled feta cheese and goes perfectly with fresh grilled fish. Traditionally made with bulgur, this variation uses spelt, which adds a mild hazelnut-like taste and extra protein, and vitamins C and K.

1 **In a small saucepan** over a high heat, bring the spelt and 750ml (1¼ pints) water to the boil; reduce the heat to medium-low and cover. Simmer for 1¼ hours, or until chewy, yet tender. Remove from the heat. Leave to stand for 10 minutes covered. Transfer to a bowl. Chill. (Note: this step can be done in advance.)

2 **Meanwhile,** whisk the lemon juice, oil, and garlic in a medium-sized bowl to blend. Add the chilled spelt. Stir with a fork.

3 **Stir in the cucumber,** spring onions, dill, and mint. Add pepper and salt to taste.

4 **Toss,** top with feta cheese, and serve. For bigger serving sizes, double the quantities.

nutritional analysis per serving: calories 180; calories from fat 90; total fat 10g; saturated fat 2.5g; cholesterol 10mg; sodium 250mg; carbohydrates 21g; dietary fibre 1g; protein 5g.

SOUPS AND SALADS

lemon bulgur salad with chickpeas and roasted peppers

serves 8

ingredients

200g (7oz) medium-grain bulgur

125ml (4fl oz) fresh lemon juice

1 large garlic clove, finely chopped

1 tin (425g/15oz) unsalted chickpeas, rinsed and drained

½ of 450g (1lb) jar roasted red peppers, drained and diced (about 115g/4oz diced)

15g (½oz) chopped fresh flat-leaf parsley leaves

2 tbsp extra-virgin olive oil

2 tbsp reduced-sodium vegetable or chicken stock

1 jalapeño pepper (with seeds), finely chopped

¼ tsp fine sea salt, or to taste

alternative grains

Use quinoa for a nice change of taste and texture for this salad.

With the flavours of chickpeas, roasted peppers, and piquant jalapeño dressing, this bulgur salad is a bit mixed up. It's part Middle Eastern, part Italian, part Mexican – but all of your taste buds will be mesmerized by the worldly mix.

1 **Place the bulgur** in a large bowl. Add 750ml (1¼ pints) boiling water and set aside for 20 minutes. Drain the bulgur well in a sieve, gently pressing out the excess liquid.

2 **Return the bulgur** to the bowl and stir in 4 tablespoons of lemon juice, the garlic, chickpeas, roasted peppers, and parsley.

3 **To make the dressing,** whisk the oil, stock, jalapeño, salt, and the remaining lemon juice in a small bowl. Drizzle the jalapeño dressing over the bulgur mixture and toss to combine.

nutritional analysis per serving: calories 210; calories from fat 40; total fat 4.5g; saturated fat 0.5g; cholesterol 0mg; sodium 370mg; carbohydrates 34g; dietary fibre 7g; protein 7g.

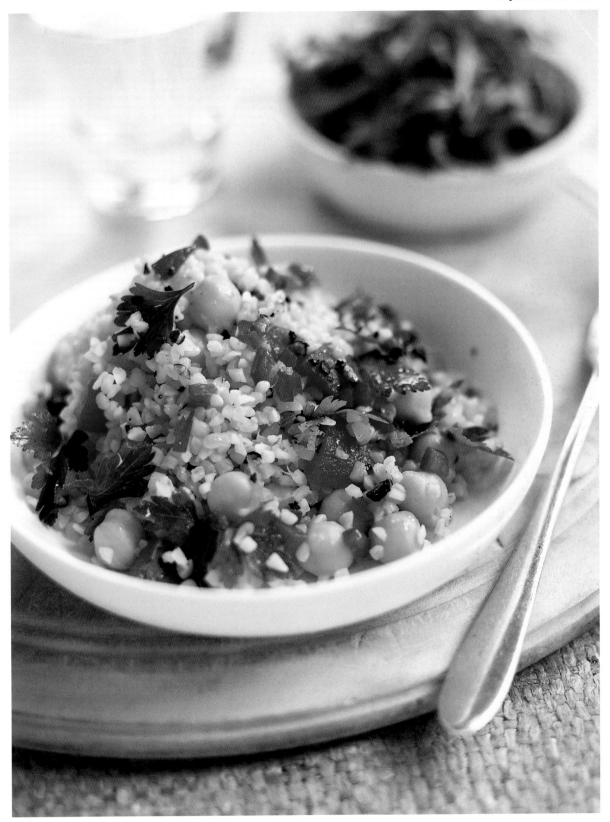

amaranth-courgette patties

serves 7
makes 14 patties

ingredients

100g (3½oz) amaranth

100g (3½oz) grated courgette, well drained (about ½ medium courgette)

45g (1½oz) finely chopped onion

35g (1¼oz) amaranth flour

1 large egg

¾ tsp garlic salt

¼ tsp hot pepper sauce, or to taste

Oil cooking spray

4 tbsp fat-free soured cream (optional)

alternative grains

Other wholegrains will work fine in place of amaranth.

If you're a fan of falafel, then you'll love these super-healthy amaranth patties. Quick and easy to prepare, these patties are the perfect party food. And with only 100 calories for two patties and lots of vitamins and minerals, they are nutritious and delicious.

1 **In a small saucepan** (preferably non-stick) over a high heat, bring the amaranth and 360ml (12fl oz) water to the boil. Reduce the heat to medium-low and cover. Simmer for 20 minutes, or until the grains are softened and the water is nearly absorbed. Remove from the heat and leave to stand, covered, for 5 minutes.

2 **Meanwhile,** in a medium-sized bowl, mix together the courgettes, onion, flour, egg, garlic salt, and hot pepper sauce. Stir in the hot cooked amaranth until well combined.

3 **Coat a large non-stick pan** with oil cooking spray and place over a medium heat. Once hot, drop the amaranth-courgette mixture by spoon onto the pan, about 2 tablespoons per patty, flattening with the back of a spoon to form round patties. Cook for 4–5 minutes per side, or until golden brown, only turning after completely done on the first side. Serve each topped with a teaspoon of fat-free soured cream, if desired.

nutritional analysis (2 patties): calories 100; calories from fat 15; total fat 2g; saturated fat 0.5g; cholesterol 30mg; sodium 110mg; carbohydrates 15g; dietary fibre 3g; protein 5g.

oatcakes with goat's cheese and prunes

serves 8
makes 16 oatcakes

ingredients

85g (3oz) rolled oats

2 tbsp unbleached
plain flour

½ tsp fine sea salt

½ tsp baking powder

2 tbsp cold unsalted
butter, cut into pieces

2–3 tbsp skimmed milk

85g (3oz) finely sliced
pitted prunes

4 tbsp pomegranate or
cranberry juice

2 tsp finely chopped fresh
thyme leaves

70g (2½oz) soft low-fat
goat's cheese

16 fresh tiny thyme sprigs

alternative grains

Boost wholegrains
further by using any
granary flour in place
of plain flour.

Oatcakes are a traditional Scottish favourite. When made with goat's cheese, prunes, and fresh herbs, they become an updated classic. Rich in fibre, oatcakes, whether served alone as a starter or over field greens as a main dish, will surely satisfy any appetite.

1 **Preheat the oven** to 190°C (375°F, gas 5). In a food processor, pulse the oats until finely chopped. Add the flour, salt, baking powder, and butter, and pulse until the mixture resembles coarse meal. Add 2 tablespoons of milk and pulse until a dough forms (you can add an extra tablespoon of milk).

2 **On a lightly floured** surface roll out the dough into a 15cm (6in) diameter round. With a 5cm (2in) round biscuit cutter, cut 16 oatcakes and put them on non-stick baking sheets 2.5cm (1in) apart. Bake in the middle of the oven for 12–15 minutes, until crisp. Transfer to a rack to cool.

3 **In a small saucepan,** combine the prunes, juice, and 2 teaspoons of thyme and simmer for 5 minutes, stirring occasionally, or until most of the liquid is evaporated. Transfer the mixture to a small bowl and leave to cool.

4 **Top each oatcake** with about half a tablespoon of prune mixture, 1 teaspoon of goat's cheese, and a thyme sprig.

nutritional analysis (2 oatcakes): calories 100; calories from fat 40; total fat 4.5g; saturated fat 2.5g; cholesterol 10mg; sodium 220mg; carbohydrates 14g; dietary fibre 2g; protein 2g.

STARTERS AND SNACKS

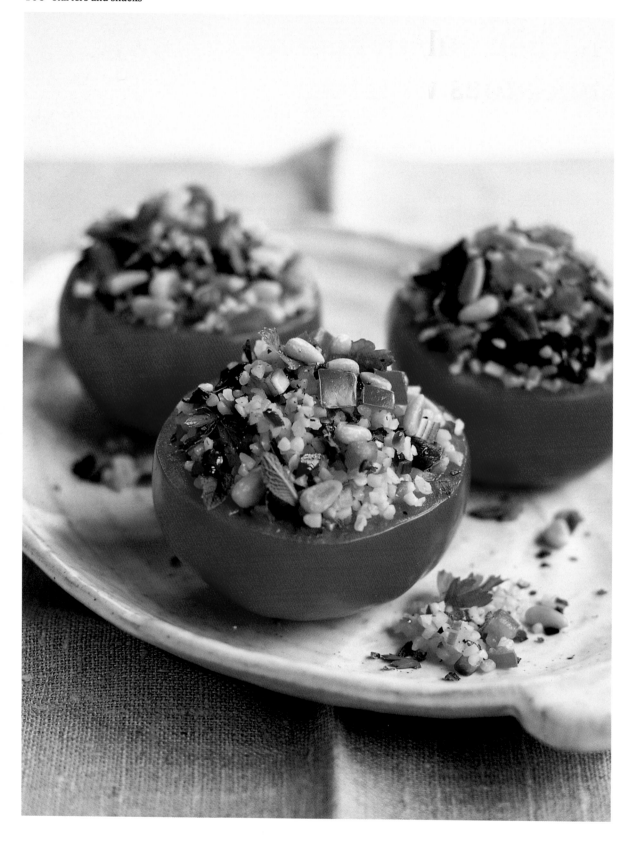

herbed bulgur-stuffed tomatoes with toasted pine nuts

serves 4

ingredients

4 large tomatoes

2 tbsp extra-virgin olive oil

1 large red onion, finely chopped

140g (5oz) medium- or coarse-grain bulgur

15g (½oz) fresh baby spinach leaves

¼ tsp fine sea salt, or to taste

¼ tsp freshly ground black pepper

45g (1½oz) pine nuts, toasted

20g (¾oz) chopped fresh parsley

3 tbsp chopped fresh mint

2 tbsp lemon juice or aged red wine vinegar

alternative grains

Quinoa or amaranth would work well in place of bulgur.

Bulgur is an incredibly healthy food and a mainstay of Middle Eastern cooking. Each serving of this dish is packed with 12 grams of fibre and 60 per cent of your daily vitamin A and C requirements, as well as iron, potassium, zinc, and magnesium.

1 **Cut off the top third** of the tomatoes. Remove the seeds and core from the top portions; dice and set aside. Scoop out the insides of the bottom portions of the tomatoes to create tomato "shells". Sit the tomato "shells" cut-side down on kitchen paper to drain.

2 **Heat the oil** in a large saucepan over a medium heat. Once hot, cook the onion in oil, stirring occasionally, for 8 minutes or until softened and lightly browned. Add the bulgur, spinach, salt, and pepper, and cook, stirring for 1 minute, or until the spinach is wilted.

3 **Add 240ml (8fl oz) water,** then remove from the heat and leave to stand, covered, for 30 minutes, or until the bulgur is softened.

4 **Stir in the pine nuts,** parsley, mint, and lemon juice or vinegar. Spoon the bulgur filling into the tomato "shells". Sprinkle with the diced tomato. Serve at room temperature.

nutritional analysis (1 stuffed tomato): calories 330; calories from fat 150; total fat 16g; saturated fat 2g; cholesterol 0mg; sodium 220mg; carbohydrates 43g; dietary fibre 12g; protein 9g.

buckwheat crêpes with goat's cheese and sun-dried tomatoes

serves 4
makes 8 crepes

ingredients

150ml (5fl oz) cold skimmed milk

1 large egg

1 tbsp unsalted butter or margarine, melted

35g (1¼oz) buckwheat flour

35g (1¼oz) unbleached plain flour

115g (4oz) soft, low-fat goat's cheese

5 sun-dried tomato halves (not oil-packed), finely chopped

¼ tsp garlic powder, or to taste

4 tsp extra-virgin olive oil

alternative grains

For a darker, earthier crepe, use 70g (2½oz) buckwheat flour instead of 35g (1¼oz) buckwheat flour plus 35g (1¼oz) plain flour.

Crêpes, when served sweet, are often eaten in the morning for breakfast. In this savoury recipe, however, crêpes are filled with goat's cheese and sun-dried tomatoes, and are transformed into a delicious late-day light bite or starter.

1 **Blend the milk,** egg, butter or margarine, and flours at high speed for 45 seconds, or until the batter is smooth. Cover the batter and refrigerate for at least 1 hour.

2 **Meanwhile,** in a small bowl stir the goat's cheese, sun-dried tomatoes, and garlic powder until well combined; chill until ready to use.

3 **Preheat the oven** to 180°C (350°F, gas 4). Add half a teaspoon of oil to a crêpe pan over a medium heat. Spoon about 2 tablespoons of batter into the pan, tilting the pan to make a thin circular crêpe. Cook for 1 minute or until the edges begin to pull away from the pan and the bottom is lightly browned. Flip the crêpe over and cook for 30 seconds, or until lightly browned. Repeat with the remaining oil and batter to make 8 crêpes.

4 **Spread the cheese** mixture on top of each crêpe. Fold the edges over, place on a large tray, and heat in the oven for 5 minutes. Serve warm.

nutritional analysis (2 crêpes): calories 210; calories from fat 120; total fat 13g; saturated fat 4g; cholesterol 60mg; sodium 310mg; carbohydrates 16g; dietary fibre 2g; protein 8g.

quinoa tuna salad sandwich on wholemeal bread

serves 6
makes 6 sandwiches

ingredients

75g (2½oz) quinoa

6 tbsp fat-free natural yoghurt

3 tbsp dairy-free mayonnaise

2 tbsp spicy Dijon mustard

Juice of 1 small or ½ large lemon (about 2 tbsp)

1 tin (170g/6 oz) solid white tuna in spring water, drained

115g (4oz) cherry tomatoes, sliced or halved

85g (3oz) finely diced onion

15g (½oz) chopped fresh flat-leaf parsley

12 slices low-calorie wholemeal bread (toasted, if desired)

alternative grains

Use amaranth instead of quinoa for a creamier texture. To reduce calories, serve quinoa-tuna mixture open face on 1 slice of low-calorie bread, or wrapped in lettuce leaves.

A tuna salad sandwich is one of the all-time classics. But you'll find a favourite new variation with this quinoa-accented version. To make your sandwich more filling, try adding alfalfa sprouts, avocado, lettuce, and extra tomato.

1 **In a small saucepan** over a high heat, bring the quinoa and 240ml (8fl oz) water to the boil. Reduce the heat to medium and cover. Simmer for 7 minutes, or until the quinoa has absorbed the water. Remove from the heat. Leave to stand for 5 minutes covered. Chill.

2 **In a large bowl,** whisk the yoghurt, mayonnaise, mustard, and lemon juice until well combined.

3 **Stir in the tuna** and quinoa until coated. Stir in the tomatoes, onions, and parsley.

4 **Serve on bread.** Slice sandwich diagonally.

nutritional analysis (1 sandwich): calories 240; calories from fat 70; total fat 8g; saturated fat 1g; cholesterol 15mg; sodium 480mg; carbohydrates 32g; dietary fibre 8g; protein 14g.

polenta-crusted oven-fried chicken fingers

serves 6
makes 12 fingers

ingredients

70g (2½oz) unbleached plain flour

1 large egg

1 large egg white

½ tsp freshly ground black pepper

¼ tsp cayenne pepper

100g (3½oz) very fine wholegrain cornmeal (polenta)

½ tsp garlic powder

450g (1lb) boneless, skinless chicken breasts, sliced diagonally into 12 long strips (fingers)

Oil cooking spray

6 tbsp honey mustard or salsa of choice

alternative grains

These "fingers" will be nice and crispy when using wholemeal breadcrumbs instead of wholegrain cornmeal (polenta). Lightly crunched wholegrain corn flakes cereal will make these even crispier.

This dish is a fun finger food and always a crunchy kid-pleaser, too. These are perfect for party snacks or served with a salad as part of a main dish. High in protein, but with a lot less fat than traditional fried chicken, this recipe gives all the taste without the guilt.

1 **Preheat the oven** to 190°C (375°F, gas 5). In a bowl add the flour. In a second bowl whisk the egg and egg whites with 2 tablespoons of cold water and the black and cayenne peppers. In a third bowl combine the cornmeal (polenta) with quarter of a teaspoon of garlic powder.

2 **Season the chicken** "fingers" with the remaining garlic powder. Dip the chicken into the flour, then the egg mixture, and then the cornmeal (polenta) mixture.

3 **Lightly coat each piece** of chicken with oil cooking spray while placing into a 22x32cm (9x13in) non-stick baking tin.

4 **Bake for 20–22 minutes,** until the internal chicken temperature reaches 76°C (170°F), turning over after 12 minutes. Serve hot or at room temperature with honey mustard or salsa of your choice.

nutritional analysis (2 chicken fingers): calories 250; calories from fat 20; total fat 2g; saturated fat 0.5g; cholesterol 80mg; sodium 230mg; carbohydrates 33g; dietary fibre 2g; protein 23g.

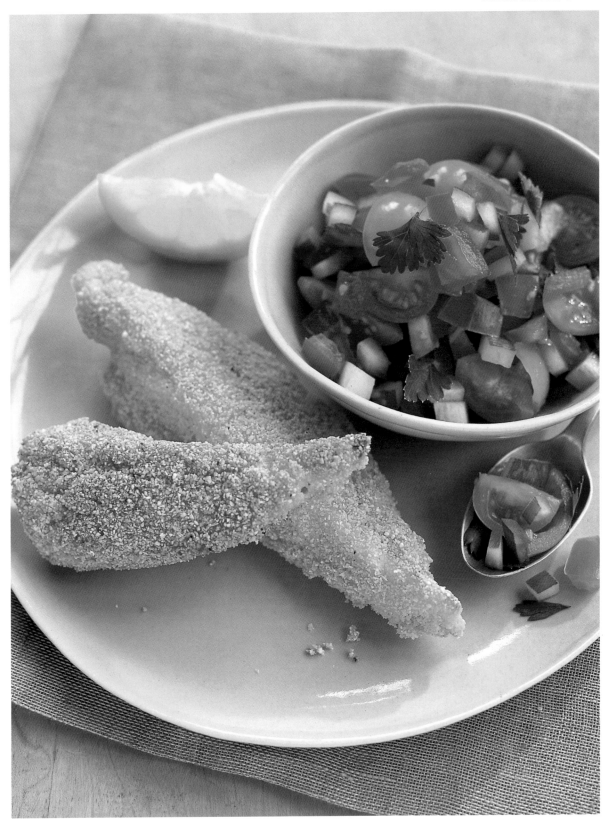

italian-inspired barley with escarole and turkey sausage

serves 4

ingredients

175g (6½oz) whole hulled barley

1 tbsp extra-virgin olive oil

170g (6oz) Italian turkey sausage, casings removed

1 head hand-torn escarole or frisée (curly endive)

2 large garlic cloves, finely chopped

240ml (8fl oz) reduced-sodium chicken stock

20g (¾oz) chopped fresh flat-leaf parsley

¼ tsp salt, or to taste

2 tbsp freshly grated Parmigiana-Reggiano cheese

alternative grains

Try any small-sized wholewheat pasta instead of barley, or serve over quinoa for another tasty option.

The barley makes this recipe really stand out from the pack. And for a zestier taste, use a spicy turkey sausage, a much healthier alternative to traditional sausage, with a lot less fat and much more fibre, folate, and vitamins.

1 **In a medium-sized saucepan** over a high heat, bring the barley and 750ml (1¼ pints) water to the boil; reduce the heat to medium-low and cover. Simmer for 45 minutes, or until chewy yet tender.

2 **Meanwhile,** add the oil to a large frying pan over a medium heat. Once the oil is hot, add the sausage and cook, breaking up clumps, for 5 minutes, or until just cooked through. Remove the sausage, leaving the fat in the frying pan.

3 **Add the escarole** and garlic to the frying pan and cook, stirring, for 3 minutes, or until the greens are wilted.

4 **Place the sausage,** barley, and stock in the saucepan. Bring to the boil over a high heat; remove from the heat.

5 **Stir in the parsley** and add salt to taste. Serve in bowls and top with cheese.

nutritional analysis per serving: calories 300; calories from fat 80; total fat 8g; saturated fat 2g; cholesterol 35mg; sodium 450mg; carbohydrates 42g; dietary fibre 10g; protein 16g.

MAIN DISHES

peppers stuffed with quinoa and minced turkey

serves 4

ingredients

100g (3½oz) quinoa

4 large red peppers

2 tsp extra-virgin olive oil

1 large red onion, chopped

3 large garlic cloves, finely chopped

360ml (12fl oz) jar tomato sauce

340g (12oz) lean minced turkey breast meat

1 large egg, beaten

20g (¾oz) chopped fresh parsley

½ tsp fine sea salt, or to taste

½ tsp ground black pepper, or to taste

alternative grains

Bulgur or brown and wild rice can be used in place of quinoa for these stuffed peppers.

In need of a rustic comfort food? These stuffed peppers are low in fat and rich in vitamins C and K, iron, zinc, and protein. For a vegetarian alternative, omit the minced turkey and use chopped aubergines or tofu instead.

1 **In a small saucepan** over a high heat, bring the quinoa and 360ml (12fl oz) water to the boil. Reduce to medium and cover. Cook for 10 minutes. Remove from the heat and leave to stand for 5 minutes covered. Transfer to a bowl. Chill.

2 **Cut off the top** 2.5cm (1in) of the peppers, discard the stems, and dice the pepper tops. Scoop out the seeds from the pepper cavities.

3 **Heat the oil** in a non-stick frying pan over a medium heat. Add the peppers, onions, and garlic and sauté for 8 minutes. Transfer to a large bowl. Add the quinoa, 120ml (4fl oz) tomato sauce, turkey, egg, parsley, salt, and pepper.

4 **Firmly stuff** and mound the turkey mixture into the pepper cavities. Stand the peppers in a single layer in a large, heavy-based pan. Pour the remaining tomato sauce and 120ml (4fl oz) water around the peppers and bring to the boil.

5 **Reduce the heat** to medium-low, cover, and simmer for 25 minutes. Spoon the sauce over each pepper. Cover and cook for 20 more minutes, until the filling is cooked. Leave to stand for 5 minutes covered. Serve with sauce over the peppers.

nutritional analysis (1 stuffed pepper): calories 390; calories from fat 90; total fat 10g; saturated fat 2g; cholesterol 85mg; sodium 490mg; carbohydrates 46g; dietary fibre 8g; protein 30g.

MAIN DISHES

sesame brown and wild rice with salmon

serves 4

ingredients

2 tsp toasted sesame oil

100g (3½oz) wild rice

100g (3½oz) brown rice

2 large garlic cloves, finely chopped

150ml (5fl oz) orange juice

4 x 85g (3oz) wild salmon fillets

2 tsp light (reduced-sodium) soy sauce

1 tsp acacia or orange blossom honey

140g (5oz) bite-sized broccoli florets

1 medium courgette, thinly sliced

2 tsp toasted sesame seeds

alternative grains

This recipe works well with amaranth, too. Barley will also add a nice, chewy texture to this dish.

Just one bite of this appealing meal will transport you to Asia. A great choice for a simple yet healthy mid-week meal, this dish is an excellent source of omega-3 fatty acids, folate, vitamins C, B_6, and B_{12}, and provides 70 per cent of your daily requirement of selenium.

1 **Add 1 teaspoon of oil** to a medium-sized saucepan over a medium heat. Once the oil is hot, add the wild rice and brown rice and cook for 1 minute. Add the garlic, 360ml (12fl oz) water, and bring to the boil over a high heat. Cover, reduce the heat to low, and simmer. After 20 minutes, add the orange juice and leave to simmer for another 20 minutes, or until the rice is tender.

2 **Preheat the oven** to 220°C (425°F, gas 7). Line a large baking sheet with baking parchment. Place the salmon on the sheet. Whisk the soy sauce and honey in a small bowl and drizzle over the salmon. Bake the salmon, uncovered, for 8–10 minutes. Remove the salmon from the oven, cover with foil, and keep warm.

3 **Heat the remaining oil** in a frying pan over a medium heat. Sauté the vegetables for 2 minutes, then cover and cook on a low heat for 5 minutes, or until crisp but still tender. Mix the vegetables with the cooked rice.

4 **Serve on a platter** topped with salmon. Sprinkle with sesame seeds.

nutritional analysis (1 salmon fillet with rice): calories 390; calories from fat 90; total fat 10g; saturated fat 1.5g; cholesterol 45mg; sodium 340mg; carbohydrates 52g; dietary fibre 3g; protein 24g.

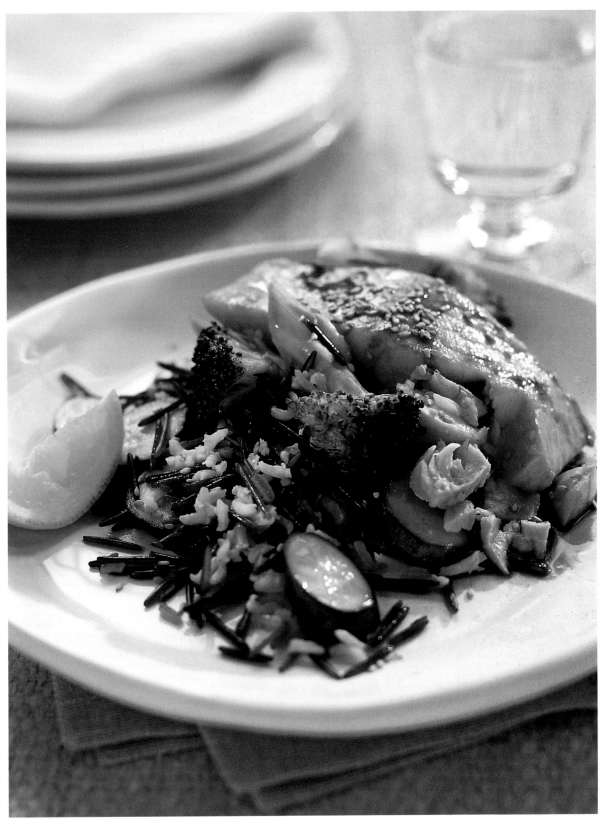

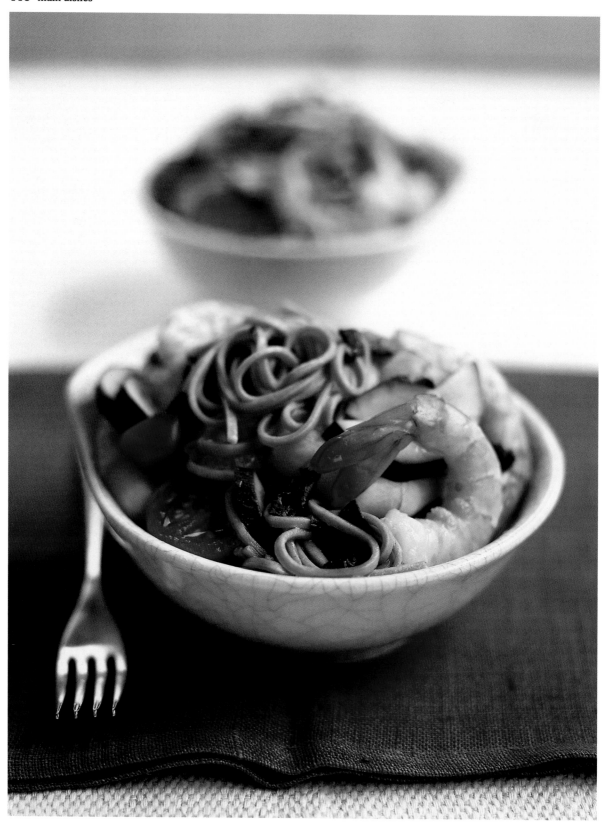

prawn soba primavera

serves 5

ingredients

340g (12oz) dry buckwheat soba noodles

2 tbsp extra-virgin olive oil

4 large garlic cloves, finely chopped

175ml (6fl oz) reduced-sodium vegetable or chicken stock

450g (1lb) precooked, deveined large prawns

20 cherry tomatoes, halved

2 medium courgettes, cut lengthways and thinly sliced

30g (1oz) chopped fresh basil

25g (scant 1oz) freshly grated Parmigiana-Reggiano cheese (optional)

alternative grains

Using udon noodles or wholewheat linguine or fettuccine will make this seem like a new dish each time it is prepared. You can also use alternative vegetables.

A much more interesting take on the typical pasta primavera, this simple dish combines the influences of Italian and Japanese cooking. With all the vegetables in this dish, prawn soba primavera is loaded with folate, vitamins A, C, and K, as well as potassium and fibre.

1 **Cook the soba noodles** in a large pan of boiling water for 4–5 minutes, or until al dente.

2 **Meanwhile,** heat the oil in a large frying pan over a medium-high heat. Add the garlic and sauté for 1 minute. Add the stock, cooked prawns, tomatoes, courgettes, and basil. Simmer for 4–5 minutes, or until the courgettes are tender and the prawns are heated through.

3 **Drain the noodles** and return to the pan. Add the prawn-vegetable mixture and toss to combine. Add salt to taste.

4 **Transfer the mixture** to a bowl and toss or sprinkle with cheese, if desired.

nutritional analysis per serving: calories 270; calories from fat 50; total fat 6g; saturated fat 1.5g; cholesterol 55mg; sodium 500mg; carbohydrates 41g; dietary fibre 1g; protein 16g.

moroccan amaranth chicken stew

serves 7

ingredients

2 tsp extra-virgin olive oil

4 x 115g (4oz) boneless, skinless chicken breasts or thighs

1 onion, diced

750ml (1¼pts) reduced-sodium chicken stock

170g (6oz) rinsed, drained, unsalted, tinned chickpeas

240ml (8fl oz) tinned, crushed tomatoes

Juice of 1 lemon (3 tbsp)

1 tsp ground cinnamon

½ tsp ground cumin

½ tsp garlic powder

170g (6oz) amaranth

30g (1oz) flaked almonds, toasted

alternative grains

Teff will provide a similar texture and a molasses-like sweetness to this thick, hearty stew.

The creamy texture of the amaranth beautifully complements this stew's spices. It's packed with goodness, too – just one portion provides 80 per cent of your iron, 50 per cent of your protein, and 25 per cent of your potassium requirements for one day.

1 **Heat the oil** in a large pan over a medium-high heat. Add the chicken and cook for 5 minutes, until brown but not cooked through. Remove to a plate.

2 **Add the onion** to the pan over a medium heat and sauté for 5 minutes. Add the stock, chickpeas, tomatoes, lemon juice, cinnamon, cumin, and garlic powder. Bring to the boil over a high heat. Stir in the amaranth. Add the chicken.

3 **Reduce the heat** to low and cover. Simmer for 25 minutes or until the chicken is cooked through. Remove from the heat and leave to stand covered for 10 minutes. Adjust the seasonings.

4 **Divide into serving bowls.** Top with almonds.

nutritional analysis per serving: calories 380; calories from fat 160; total fat 17g; saturated fat 4g; cholesterol 60mg; sodium 320mg; carbohydrates 32g; dietary fibre 4g; protein 25g.

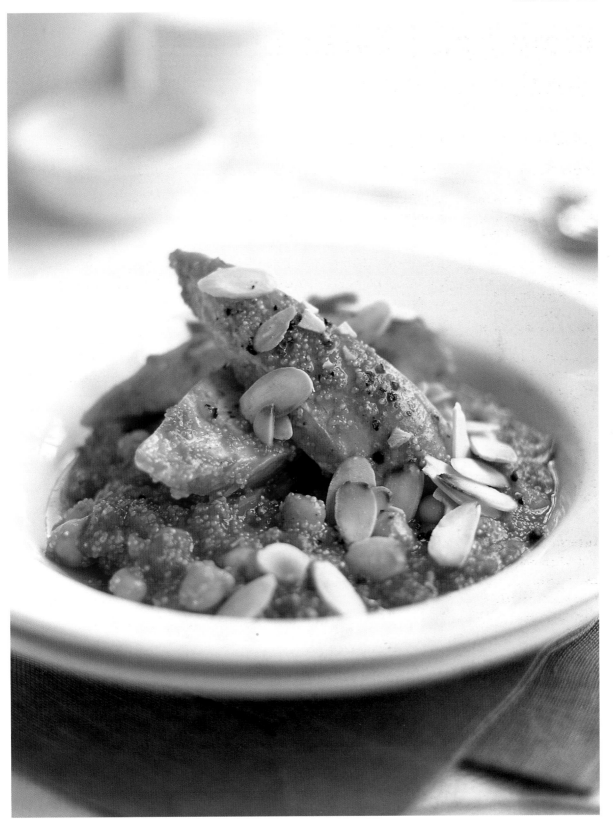

red kidney beans and spelt

serves 6

ingredients

300g (10½oz) small dry
red kidney beans, rinsed,
soaked in water in
refrigerator overnight,
drained

1.4 litres (2½pts)
reduced-sodium chicken
or vegetable stock

100g (3½oz) smoked
ham, finely chopped

1 large onion, chopped

1 large green pepper,
chopped

30g (1oz) chopped fresh
flat-leaf parsley

4 large garlic cloves,
finely chopped

1 bay leaf

½ tsp hot pepper sauce,
or to taste

55g (2oz) spelt

15g (½oz) finely snipped
fresh chives

alternative grains

This is also delicious
made with brown rice.

*The spelt and kidney beans in this Cajun-inspired dish are packed with
protein and are low in fat, too. If you haven't tried spelt before, the
cooked kernels have a sweet, nutty taste and a rice-like texture. Serve
with steamed peppers or other vegetables for a delicious meal.*

1 **Into a large pan** add the beans, stock, ham, onion, green pepper, half
the parsley, garlic, bay leaves, and hot pepper sauce. Place over a
medium heat and stir. Cook, uncovered, for 1 hour, stirring occasionally.
Cover and cook for 30 more minutes, until the beans are tender and the
liquid is absorbed. Remove the bay leaf. If necessary, add salt to taste.

2 **In a medium-sized saucepan** over a high heat, bring the spelt and
900ml (1½ pints) water to the boil; reduce to medium-low and cover.
Simmer for 1½ hours or until tender. Remove from the heat and leave
to stand for 10 minutes covered.

3 **Serve the red kidney beans** over the spelt. Sprinkle with chives and
the remaining parsley.

nutritional analysis per serving: calories 340; calories from fat 25; total fat 3g;
saturated fat 1g; cholesterol 55mg; sodium 320mg; carbohydrates 55g;
dietary fibre 15g; protein 25g.

sweet tomato-glazed veggie loaf

serves 4

ingredients

340g (12oz) packet vegetarian minced beef

1 medium red onion, grated

1 large egg, slightly beaten

1 large egg white, slightly beaten

25g (scant 1oz) rolled oats

6 tbsp tomato ketchup

2 tsp spicy brown mustard

1 tsp finely chopped fresh thyme leaves, plus additional sprigs for garnish, if desired

½ tsp garlic powder, or to taste

½ tsp freshly ground black pepper

⅛ tsp ground cinnamon (optional)

alternative grains

Cooked, chilled amaranth or teff is a nice alternative to oats in this recipe.

An exciting twist on traditional meatloaf – there is actually no meat in this dish at all. Moist and bursting with nutrients, this veggie loaf is a rich source of B vitamins, especially B_{12}, as well as zinc and iron.

1 **Preheat the oven** to 200°C (400°F, gas 6). Combine the vegetarian minced beef, onion, egg and egg white, oats, 4 tablespoons of ketchup, mustard, thyme, garlic powder, pepper, and, if using, cinnamon.

2 **On a 22x33cm** (9x13in) non-stick baking tin, form the meatloaf mixture into a loaf shape, about 17x11cm (7x4½in). Brush the remaining ketchup over the loaf.

3 **Bake for 40 minutes,** or until cooked through. (Note: unlike a traditional meatloaf, this will still be quite moist when cooked.) Leave to stand for 10 minutes before slicing.

4 **Cut into 4 slices.** If desired, garnish with thyme sprigs.

nutritional analysis (1 slice): calories 180; calories from fat 15; total fat 2g; saturated fat 0g; cholesterol 55mg; sodium 730mg; carbohydrates 20g; dietary fibre 6g; protein 20g.

MAIN DISHES

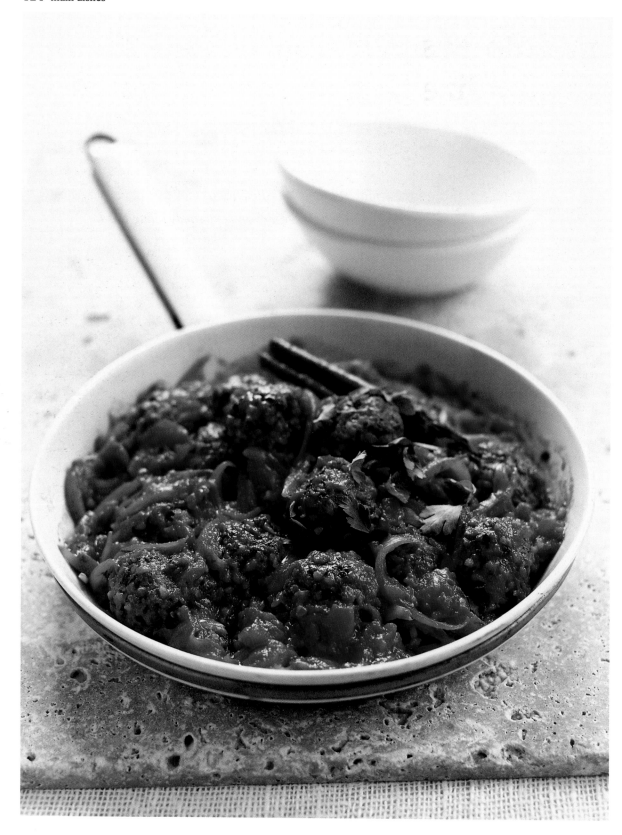

middle-eastern meatballs with caramelized onion tomato sauce

serves 6
makes 18 meatballs

ingredients

450g (1lb) lean minced beef or lamb

45g (1½oz) finely chopped fresh parsley, plus additional for garnish, if desired

15g (½oz) finely chopped fresh mint

70g (2½oz) medium-grain bulgur

4 large garlic cloves, finely chopped

¼ tsp fine sea salt

½ tsp freshly ground black pepper

1 tbsp extra-virgin olive oil

1 large white onion, thinly sliced

125ml (4fl oz) dry red wine

1 tin (360ml / 12fl oz) organic diced tomatoes with juice

1 cinnamon stick

alternative grains

For a change, try rolled oats instead of bulgur, and use ground turkey to reduce the fat content.

Give your traditional meatball recipe a nutritious kick by adding bulgur wheat, a staple in Middle Eastern cooking. These meatballs are so delicious, they can be eaten just as they are, or paired with wholewheat pasta for a healthy and extremely filling meal.

1 **In a large bowl,** combine the meat, parsley, mint, bulgur, half of the finely chopped garlic, 4 tablespoons of water, and salt and pepper.

2 **Shape the mixture** into 18 meatballs, about 2 tablespoons per meatball. Place on a plate, cover, and chill.

3 **Heat the oil** in a large frying pan over a medium-high heat. Sauté the onion for 5 minutes. Add the remaining garlic and sauté for 30 seconds. Add the wine and cook for 1 minute. Stir in the tomatoes and cinnamon stick.

4 **Add the meatballs** to the frying pan. Add 120ml (4fl oz) water, bring to the boil, and reduce the heat to medium-low. Cover and simmer for 20 minutes. Turn the meatballs over and continue cooking uncovered for 10 more minutes, or until the sauce has thickened. Remove the cinnamon stick.

nutritional analysis (3 meatballs): calories 260; calories from fat 90; total fat 10g; saturated fat 3g; cholesterol 50mg; sodium 330mg; carbohydrates 16g; dietary fibre 3g; protein 24g.

spinach and goat's cheese wholegrain pizza

serves 6

ingredients

1 sachet (7g/¼oz) easy-blend dried yeast

About 550g (1¼lb) wholegrain flour plus extra for kneading

Oil cooking spray

1½ tbsp extra-virgin olive oil

¼ tsp fine sea salt

90g (3¼oz) baby spinach leaves

1 tbsp fresh lemon juice

115g (4oz) soft, low-fat goat's cheese, crumbled

2 tbsp chopped fresh basil

¼ tsp freshly ground black pepper

¼ tsp garlic powder, or to taste

alternative grains

Try this recipe with kamut flour for a buttery flavoured crust.

This dish not only tastes great, but it is also loaded with vitamins and minerals. The best part of this pizza, though, is the crust, which has a rich, nutty flavour and lots of fibre. If you're feeling adventurous, try topping it with other vegetables, too, such as rocket or broccoli.

1 **In a medium-sized bowl,** combine the yeast and 315ml (11fl oz) warm water. Leave to stand for 10 minutes, or until the yeast softens. In a large bowl, add the flour. Make a well in the centre and pour the yeast mixture into the well. Stir vigorously with a spoon until smooth. Place the dough on a lightly floured surface. Knead by hand for 8 minutes, or until smooth and slightly springy. Rub the dough with half a tablespoon of oil. Place in a large bowl. Cover tightly with cling film and let the dough rise for 1½ hours.

2 **Preheat the oven** to 240°C (475°F, gas 9). Coat a large ovenproof non-stick tin or pizza tin with oil cooking spray. Add salt to the dough and knead to distribute the salt and form a dough ball. Press the dough ball into a 35cm (14in) round in the tin.

3 **In a medium-sized bowl,** toss the spinach with the remaining oil and the lemon juice. Top the pizza with the spinach and crumbled goat's cheese. Bake for 10 minutes, or until the pizza dough is brown and crisp.

4 **Remove** from the oven. Top with basil, pepper, and garlic powder.

nutritional analysis (1 slice): calories 330; calories from fat 70; total fat 8g; saturated fat 2g; cholesterol 5mg; sodium 200mg; carbohydrates 53g; dietary fibre 9g; protein 12g.

MAIN DISHES

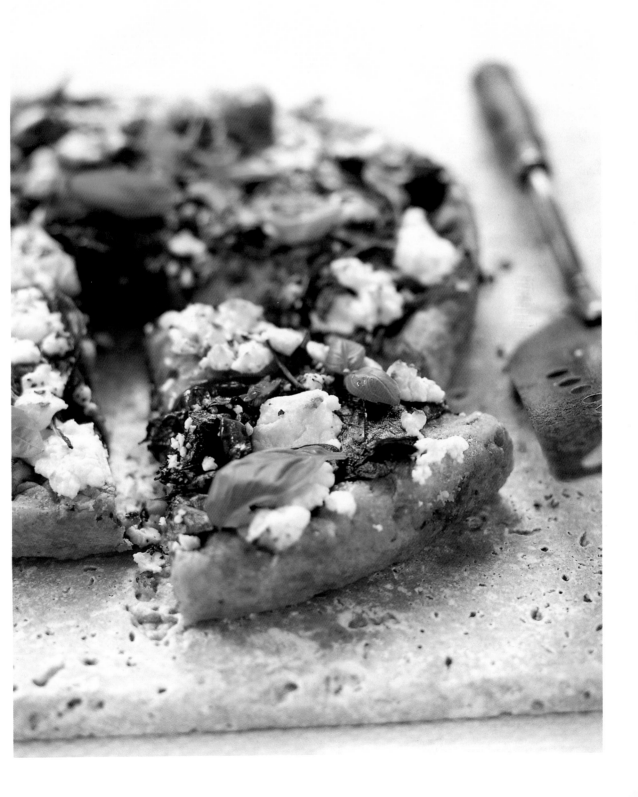

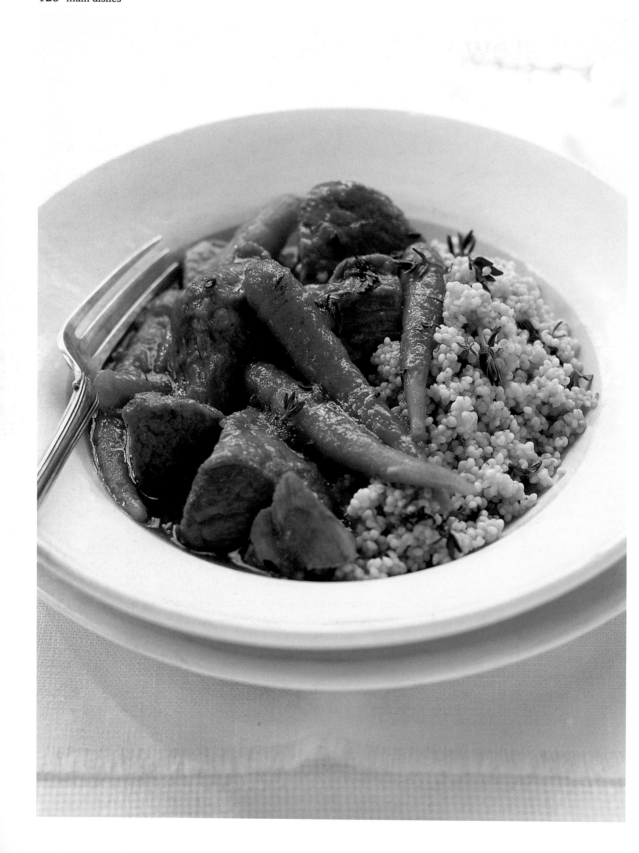

veal stew with millet, baby carrots, and thyme

serves 4

ingredients

1½ tbsp extra-virgin olive oil

680g (1½lb) veal stewing meat, cut into cubes

1 large red onion, cut into large dice

½ tsp freshly ground black pepper

475ml (16fl oz) reduced-sodium beef stock

1 tbsp finely chopped fresh thyme leaves

450g (1lb) baby carrots

100g (3½oz) millet

315ml (11fl oz) reduced-sodium vegetable, chicken, or beef stock

alternative grains

Amaranth, quinoa, or fine bulgur are ideal alternatives to millet in this stew.

This is one of the simplest stew recipes you'll find. What's more, this recipe is not only high in protein, but the carrots it contains provide 500 per cent of your daily requirements for vitamin A. It's also high in B vitamins and a range of minerals.

1 **Preheat the oven** to 180°C (350°F, gas 4). Heat the oil in a casserole or large ovenproof pot over a medium-high heat. Add the veal, onions, and pepper. Sauté for 7 minutes or until the veal is just cooked through.

2 **Mix in the beef stock** and 2 teaspoons of thyme. Bring to a simmer. Cover and roast in the oven for 30 minutes. Stir in the carrots. Cover the casserole and roast for an additional 1½ hours, or until the veal is tender. Adjust the seasonings.

3 **Place a small saucepan** over a medium-high heat. Add the millet and stir for 3 minutes, or until the millet begins to turn golden brown. Add the stock and bring to the boil. Reduce to medium-low and cover. Simmer for 18 minutes, or until the millet is softened and the liquid is absorbed. Remove from the heat. Stir in the remaining thyme. Leave to stand, covered, for 5 minutes.

4 **To serve,** ladle the stew over the millet in four shallow soup bowls.

nutritional analysis per serving: calories 370; calories from fat 90; total fat 9g; saturated fat 2.5g; cholesterol 90mg; sodium 390mg; carbohydrates 41g; dietary fibre 4g; protein 28g.

barley risotto with vine-ripened tomatoes and feta

SIDE DISHES

serves 6

ingredients

85g (3oz) whole hulled barley

2 tbsp extra-virgin olive oil

45g (1½oz) chopped shallots

125ml (4fl oz) dry red wine

475ml (16fl oz) reduced-sodium chicken or vegetable stock

1 tsp margarine or unsalted butter

¼ tsp fine sea salt, or to taste

¼ tsp freshly ground black pepper, or to taste

1 large vine-ripened tomato, seeded and finely diced

25g (scant 1oz) crumbled feta cheese

15g (½oz) finely chopped fresh basil (optional)

alternative grains

As a twist to this recipe, try farro, a grain that has garnered high culinary acclaim in Italy. It will provide a similar texture to barley, but adjust the simmering time.

For a taste of the Mediterranean, try this delicious, yet highly nutritious, twist on traditional risotto. This side dish is extremely rich in fibre, as well as essential vitamins and minerals. Team with Veal stew with millet, baby carrots, and thyme (see pp128–29) for a simple, tasty meal.

1 **In a large saucepan** over a high heat, bring the barley, 1 tablespoon of oil, and 360ml (12fl oz) water to the boil; reduce the heat to medium-low and cover. Simmer for 55 minutes, or until the barley is tender. Drain.

2 **Add the remaining oil** to a medium-sized saucepan over a medium heat. Add the shallots and sauté for 1 minute. Add the strained barley and wine. Cook for 3 minutes, or until almost all the liquid evaporates, stirring frequently.

3 **Increase the heat** to medium-high. Add 240ml (8fl oz) stock and cook, stirring frequently, for 5 minutes, or until the liquid is absorbed. Add the remaining stock and cook, stirring frequently, for 5 minutes, or until the liquid is absorbed.

4 **Remove from the heat** and stir in the margarine or butter. Add salt and pepper to taste. Fold in the tomatoes. Top with feta. If desired, garnish with finely chopped fresh basil.

nutritional analysis per serving: calories 170; calories from fat 70; total fat 8g; saturated fat 2g; cholesterol 15mg; sodium 240mg; carbohydrates 19g; dietary fibre 3g; protein 6g.

millet mashers (mock mashed potatoes)

serves 10

ingredients

2 tsp margarine or unsalted butter

1 tsp rapeseed or vegetable oil

Florets of 1 head cauliflower, chopped

200g (7oz) millet

4 large garlic cloves, peeled

1 tsp fine sea salt, or to taste

15g (½oz) snipped fresh chives

alternative grains

Using amaranth in this recipe will provide a creamier consistency.

Surprise your dinner guests with this modern re-working of a classic side dish. It looks a bit like mashed potatoes, and is just as filling, but has a unique taste and texture of its own. What's more, it's also a lot healthier than white potatoes.

1 **Add the margarine** or butter and the oil to a large saucepan over a medium-high heat. Once the butter or margarine melts, add the cauliflower and sauté for 3 minutes. Add the millet and sauté for 3 more minutes, or until lightly browned.

2 **Carefully add** 1.7 litres (3 pints) water, the garlic cloves and salt, and bring to the boil over a high heat. Cover, reduce the heat to low, and simmer for 1 hour, or just until no liquid remains.

3 **Pour the mixture** into a bowl and mash with a potato masher. Adjust the seasonings.

4 **Stir in or top** with chives.

nutritional analysis per serving: calories 150; calories from fat 25; total fat 2.5g; saturated fat 1g; cholesterol 0mg; sodium 260mg; carbohydrates 27g; dietary fibre 5g; protein 5g.

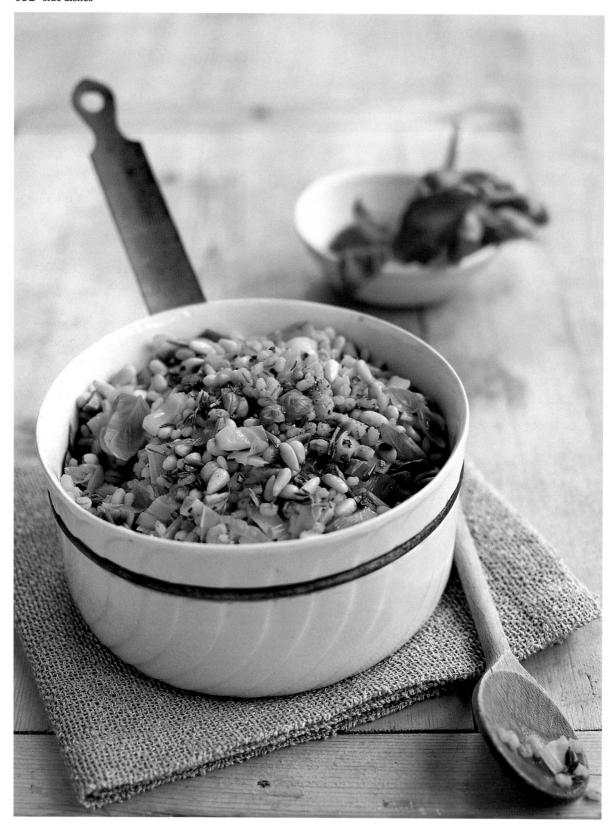

barley with leeks and fennel

serves 6

ingredients

1 tbsp rapeseed or vegetable oil

2 leeks (white and pale green parts only), chopped

1 fennel bulb, finely chopped

280g (10oz) whole hulled barley

1 litre (1¾pts) reduced-sodium chicken stock

Few saffron threads

25g (scant 1oz) freshly grated Parmigiana-Reggiano cheese

30g (1oz) chopped fresh basil

1 tsp finely chopped fresh thyme leaves

½ tsp freshly ground black pepper, or to taste

3 tbsp pine nuts, toasted

alternative grains

Small-sized wholewheat pasta will be wonderful instead of barley. Cooking time and amount of stock will need to be adjusted.

This barley recipe is healthy enough to prepare as often as you like. The precious spice saffron takes it to an aromatic level of its own. And, if you're looking to boost your fibre intake, especially soluble fibre, then this dish is the one for you.

1 **Add the oil** to a large saucepan over a medium heat. Once the oil is hot, sauté the leeks and fennel for 8 minutes, or until tender.

2 **Stir in the barley,** stock, and saffron and bring to the boil over a high heat. Reduce the heat to medium-low, cover, and simmer for 90 minutes, or until the barley is tender.

3 **Stir in the cheese,** three-quarters of the basil, and the thyme. Add pepper to taste.

4 **Serve.** Top with the remaining basil and sprinkle with pine nuts.

nutritional analysis per serving: calories 300; calories from fat 80; total fat 8g; saturated fat 1.5g; cholesterol 20mg; sodium 180mg; carbohydrates 47g; dietary fibre 10g; protein 12g.

SIDE DISHES

citrus-pistachio spelt pilaf

serves 4

ingredients

1 tsp extra-virgin olive oil

1 tsp margarine or
unsalted butter

2 large shallots, finely
chopped

55g (2oz) spelt

45g (1½ oz) unsalted,
shelled pistachio nuts,
chopped, plus extra
for garnish

240ml (8fl oz) reduced-
sodium chicken stock

4 tbsp fresh orange juice

Juice of 1 lemon (3 tbsp
juice)

¼ tsp fine sea salt,
or to taste

⅛ tsp white pepper,
or to taste

alternative grains

You'll particularly enjoy
the crunch of the
pistachio nuts in this pilaf
when using a grain that's
softer when cooked, such
as long-grain brown rice.
Cooking time and liquid
will need to be adjusted.

This is a brilliant pilaf bursting with zesty citrus flavours. The pistachios complement spelt's nutty flavour, creating a delicious dish that is rich in vitamin C, packed with riboflavin, and perfect for when you're in need of an energy boost. Serve with grilled chicken or seafood.

1 **Heat the oil** and margarine or butter in a large saucepan over a medium heat. Once the butter melts, add the shallots and sauté for 2 minutes. Add the spelt and half of the pistachio nuts and sauté for 1 more minute.

2 **Increase the heat** to high. Carefully add 360ml (12fl oz) water, stock, and juices and bring to the boil.

3 **Reduce the heat** to medium-low. Cover and simmer for 1¼ hours, or until the liquid is absorbed and the spelt is chewy yet tender. Remove from the heat. Leave to stand, covered, for 10 minutes.

4 **Add salt and pepper** to taste. Garnish the spelt with a few pistachio nuts.

nutritional analysis per serving: calories 190; calories from fat 60; total fat 6g; saturated fat 1g; cholesterol 5mg; sodium 290mg; carbohydrates 32g; dietary fibre 1g; protein 7g.

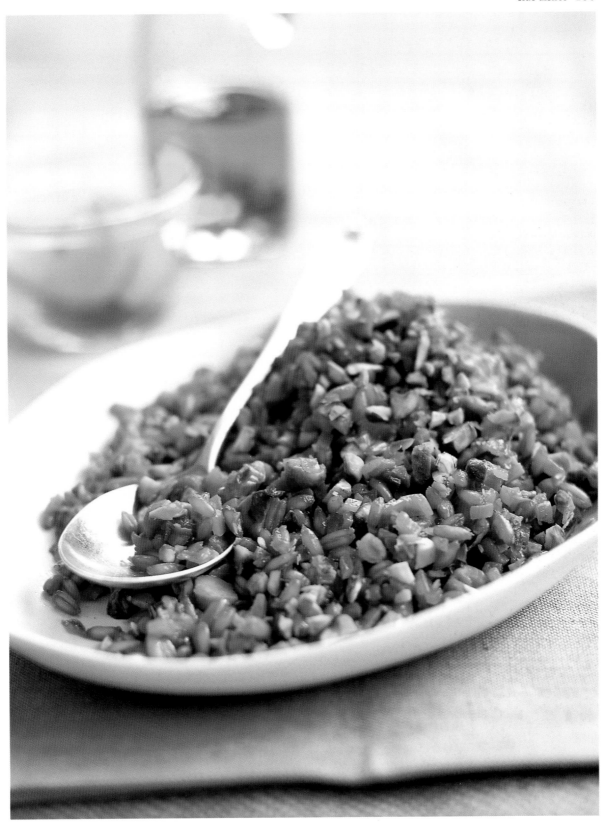

sweet pepper, sorghum, and pine nut pilaf

serves 6

ingredients

250g (8½oz) sorghum

1 tbsp extra-virgin olive oil

1 small or ½ large red onion, finely chopped

120ml (4fl oz) reduced-sodium vegetable or chicken stock

Juice of 1 small lemon (2 tbsp)

1 large red or orange pepper, finely diced

15g (½oz) chopped fresh basil

2 tbsp finely snipped fresh chives

30g (1oz) pine nuts, toasted

½ tsp fine sea salt, or to taste

¼ tsp freshly ground black pepper, or to taste

alternative grains

If you're having trouble obtaining sorghum, prepare with quinoa for an easy substitution.

A colourful side dish that's quick to make, this recipe is delicious served hot or cold. It's highly nutritious and a great source of vitamin C. Look for sorghum in speciality food shops that carry African and Indian products, or try preparing this pilaf with an alternative grain instead.

1 **In a medium-sized saucepan** over a high heat, bring the sorghum and 600ml (1 pint) water to the boil; reduce to medium and cover. Cook for 12 minutes, or until tender. Remove from the heat and leave to stand for 5 minutes covered.

2 **Meanwhile,** add the oil to a large non-stick frying pan over a medium heat. Once the oil is hot, sauté the onion for 5 minutes, or until softened.

3 **Stir in the stock,** lemon juice, and pepper. Continue cooking for 5 minutes. (Note: some liquid will still remain.)

4 **Stir in the cooked sorghum**. Once the sorghum is hot and the mixture is well combined, remove from the heat.

5 **Stir in the basil** and chives. Sprinkle with pine nuts, salt, and pepper.

nutritional analysis per serving: calories 220; calories from fat 60; total fat 7g; saturated fat 0.5g; cholesterol 0mg; sodium 240mg; carbohydrates 35g; dietary fibre 2g; protein 5g.

garlic-ginger kale with quinoa and sesame

serves 6

ingredients

475ml (16fl oz) reduced-sodium chicken or vegetable stock

140g (5oz) quinoa

1 large bunch kale, very thinly sliced (thick stems discarded)

1 tbsp grated fresh ginger

1 large garlic clove, finely chopped

1 tbsp toasted sesame oil

1 tbsp rice vinegar

1 tbsp acacia or orange blossom honey

1½ tsp reduced-sodium soy sauce

1 tbsp toasted sesame seeds

alternative grains

In place of quinoa, try wild or brown rice. Cooking times will need to be adjusted depending on which grain you choose.

This garlic and ginger infused side dish has the winning combination of being incredibly flavourful and easy to prepare. It's also fantastic for your health, with kale providing calcium, folic acid, iron, potassium, as well as a range of antioxidants.

1 **Bring the stock to the boil** in a casserole or large saucepan over a high heat. Add the quinoa, kale, ginger, and garlic. Don't stir. Cover, reduce the heat to low, and cook for 15 minutes. Remove from the heat and leave to stand, covered, for 5 minutes.

2 **In a small bowl,** whisk the oil, vinegar, honey, and soy sauce. Drizzle over the quinoa-kale mixture and stir well.

3 **Serve hot.** Sprinkle with sesame seeds.

nutritional analysis per serving: calories 210; calories from fat 50; total fat 6g; saturated fat 1g; cholesterol 10mg; sodium 180mg; carbohydrates 33g; dietary fibre 4g; protein 9g.

SIDE DISHES

pepper, courgette, and buckwheat sauté

serves 8

ingredients

180g (6½oz) buckwheat groats

2 tbsp extra-virgin olive oil

750ml (1¼pts) reduced-sodium vegetable or chicken stock

1 large red onion, chopped

2 large garlic cloves, finely chopped

1 large red pepper, chopped

1 large yellow pepper, chopped

1 medium courgette, cut lengthways and thinly sliced

1 tsp finely chopped fresh oregano, plus additional leaves for garnish, if desired

¼ tsp fine sea salt, or to taste

½ tsp freshly ground black pepper, or to taste

alternative grains

If buckwheat isn't to your liking, enjoy this dish with wholewheat couscous or bulgur.

This mouthwatering sauté is a healthier version of vegetable stir-fried rice. It's so moist, consider moulding individual portions. All of the peppers in this dish actually give you 150 per cent of your daily vitamin C requirement.

1 **Toast the buckwheat** in a large saucepan over a medium-high heat, stirring constantly for 4 minutes, or until richly fragrant. Stir in 1 tablespoon of oil. Once the buckwheat is coated, carefully add the stock and bring to the boil. Reduce the heat to low, cover, and simmer for 10 minutes. Remove from the heat and keep covered for 10 minutes.

2 **Heat the remaining oil** in a large non-stick frying pan over a medium heat. Sauté the onion, garlic, and peppers for 5 minutes. Add the courgette and oregano and sauté for 5 more minutes, until the vegetables are softened.

3 **Stir the buckwheat** into the vegetables in the pan until well combined. Add salt and pepper to taste. If desired, garnish with oregano leaves.

nutritional analysis per serving: calories 180; calories from fat 40; total fat 4.5g; saturated fat 0.5g; cholesterol 0mg; sodium 280mg; carbohydrates 29g; dietary fibre 4g; protein 6g.

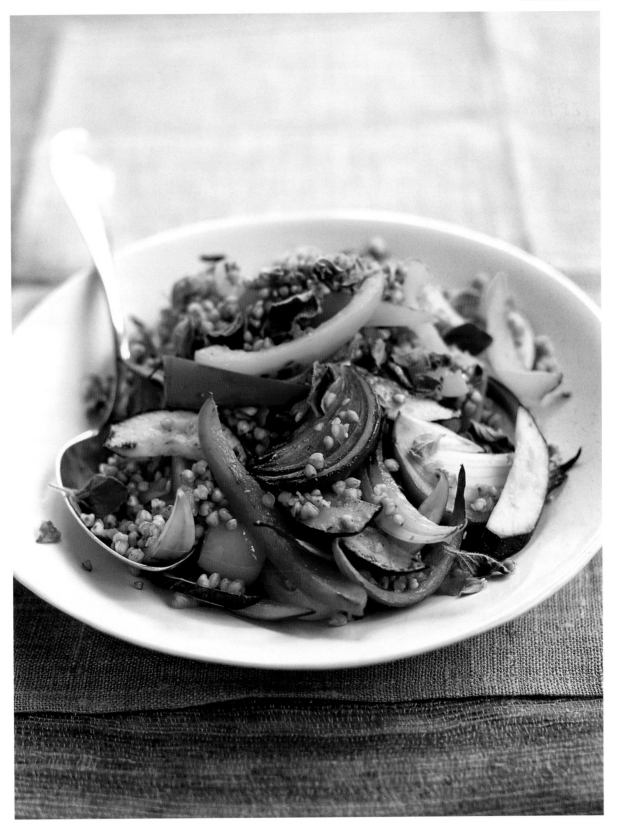

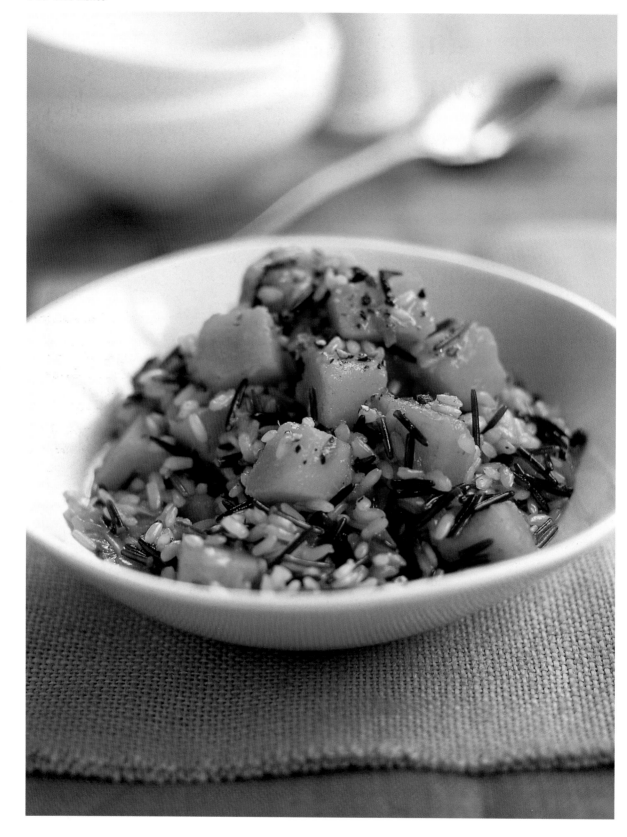

curried squash risotto with brown and wild rice

serves 6

ingredients

½ of a medium-sized butternut squash, peeled and seeded

1.5 litres (2¾pts) reduced-sodium chicken stock

1 tbsp extra-virgin olive oil

1 medium onion, chopped

200g (7oz) long-grain brown rice

100g (3½oz) wild rice

2 large garlic cloves, finely chopped

1½ tsp curry powder

Juice of 1 lime (2 tbsp), or to taste

4 tsp unsalted butter or margarine (optional)

alternative grains

Try with all brown rice instead of a mixture of brown and wild rice.

While classic risotto is made with Arborio rice, this one uses brown and wild rice. This variation not only increases the fibre content, but also, the squash in one serving provides a full day's worth of vitamin A. Try this delicious rice dish as an accompaniment to grilled chicken.

1 **Halve the squash** lengthways. Remove the skin with a vegetable peeler and remove the seeds from only one half. Dice.

2 **In a large saucepan** over a medium-low heat, bring the stock to a simmer.

3 **Heat the oil** separately in a large pan over a medium-high heat. Sauté the squash and onion for 8 minutes, or until lightly caramelized. Add the brown and wild rice, garlic, and curry powder and cook, stirring, for 1 minute. Reduce the heat to medium. Carefully stir in 125ml (4fl oz) simmering stock and cook, stirring frequently, until the stock is absorbed. Continue simmering and adding stock 125ml (4fl oz) at a time, stirring constantly, making sure each addition is absorbed before adding the next. (Note: the risotto will take about 50 minutes.)

4 **Stir in the lime juice** and simmer, stirring, for 1 minute. Serve the risotto immediately. If desired, top each with a teaspoon of butter.

nutritional analysis per serving: calories 250; calories from fat 30; total fat 3.5g; saturated fat 0.5g; cholesterol 0mg; sodium 610mg; carbohydrates 46g; dietary fibre 4g; protein 9g.

southwestern-style american cornbread

makes 1 loaf – 20 slices

ingredients

Oil cooking spray

115g (4oz) margarine or unsalted butter, melted

200g (7oz) granulated sugar

4 large eggs

4 tbsp fat-free evaporated milk

1 x 280g (10oz) packet frozen sweetcorn, thawed and drained, or 300g (10½oz) fresh cooked sweetcorn kernels

70g (2½oz) grated Gouda cheese

140g (5oz) very fine wholegrain cornmeal (polenta)

140g (5oz) unbleached plain flour

1 tbsp plus 1 tsp baking powder

½ tsp fine sea salt

alternative grains

Consider using a mixture of flours such as wholemeal, millet, amaranth, or buckwheat.

Cornbread is a truly American food, particularly of the southern states. To spice up this mellow recipe, give it a TexMex makeover by adding finely chopped jalapeño peppers to the mixture. To avoid skin irritation, be sure to wear rubber gloves when handling the peppers.

1 **Preheat the oven** to 150°C (300°F, gas 2). Lightly coat a 22x32cm (9x13in) non-stick baking tin with oil cooking spray.

2 **In a large bowl,** beat the melted margarine or butter and sugar. Beat in the eggs one at a time. Blend in the milk, sweetcorn, and cheese.

3 **In a separate bowl**, combine the cornmeal (polenta), flour, baking powder, and salt. Add the cornmeal (polenta) mixture to the sweetcorn mixture and blend until well combined.

4 **Pour the mixture** into the prepared tin. Bake for 1 hour, or until a cocktail stick inserted comes out clean. (Note: the sweetcorn kernels will settle to the bottom of the bread during baking.) Remove the tin to a rack to cool.

nutritional analysis (1 slice): calories 170; calories from fat 60; total fat 7g; saturated fat 4g; cholesterol 60mg; sodium 210mg; carbohydrates 23g; dietary fibre 1g; protein 4g.

soft rye bread

**serves 24
makes 2 loaves –
12 slices each**

ingredients

About 500g (1lb, 2oz) unbleached plain flour plus extra for dusting

50g (1¾oz) dark brown sugar

2 sachets active dry yeast (14g/½oz)

3 tsp whole caraway seeds

1½ tsp fine sea salt

1 tsp grated orange zest (optional)

2 tbsp rapeseed or vegetable oil

280g (10oz) dark rye flour

Oil cooking spray

1 egg white

alternative grains

Consider using a mixture of flours to create granary bread. Or, simply go a little heavier on the rye flour.

Rye bread is so healthy and tasty that it should be a staple of any kitchen. This delicious version is made the old-fashioned way: no bread machine required. Plus, this recipe has the best of both bread worlds – half rye and half wheat.

1 **In a large bowl,** combine 280g (10oz) plain flour, brown sugar, yeast (not dissolved), 2 teaspoons of caraway seeds, salt, and, if using, orange zest. Gradually add 475ml (16fl oz) warm water and oil to the flour mixture and beat with an electric mixer for 2 minutes at medium speed. Add 70g (2½oz) plain flour and beat for 2 minutes at high speed. Stir in the rye flour and just enough plain flour to make soft dough.

2 **Knead the dough** on a lightly floured surface for 8 minutes, or until elastic. Cover and leave to rest for 10 minutes. Divide the dough in half and shape each into a loaf. Place on a large non-stick baking sheet lightly coated with oil cooking spray. Cover loosely with clingfilm or foil that has been coated in cooking spray and leave to rise in a warm, draught-free place for 1 hour, until doubled in size.

3 **Preheat the oven** to 200°C (400°F, gas 6). With a knife make 6 slashes on top of each loaf. In a small bowl, whisk the egg white with 1 tablespoon of cold water. Brush the egg white mixture over the loaves. Sprinkle with the remaining caraway seeds.

4 **Bake for 30 minutes,** or until cooked. Remove the loaves and leave to cool on a rack.

nutritional analysis (1 slice): calories 120; calories from fat 15; total fat 1.5g; saturated fat 0g; cholesterol 0mg; sodium 150mg; carbohydrates 23g; dietary fibre 2g; protein 3g.

nutty millet banana bread

**serves 24
makes 1 loaf – 24
thin slices**

ingredients

115g (4oz) unsalted
butter, melted

200g (7oz) granulated
sugar

2 large eggs, well beaten

140g (5oz) unbleached
plain flour

100g (3½oz) wholemeal
flour

1 tsp bicarbonate of soda

¼ tsp fine sea salt

100g (3½oz) millet

4 large fully ripened
bananas, mashed

2 tsp pure vanilla extract

45g (1½oz) chopped
walnuts, toasted

Oil cooking spray

alternative grains

Using rolled oats instead
of millet will give this
bread a smooth,
comforting texture.

This banana bread is nutritious enough for breakfast, but sweet enough for dessert. The millet gives this moist treat a unique, almost candy-like crunchiness. This bread is delicious freshly baked or topped with low-sugar jam.

1 **Preheat the oven** to 180°C (350°F, gas 4). In a large mixing bowl, cream the melted butter and sugar with an electric mixer. Add the beaten eggs and blend well.

2 **In a separate bowl,** sift the flours, bicarbonate of soda, and salt. Add the sifted dry ingredients to the butter mixture. Blend on low speed, until just combined.

3 **Add the millet,** mashed bananas, vanilla extract, and nuts to the mixture and stir until just mixed.

4 **Coat a non-stick loaf tin** with oil cooking spray. Pour the mixture into the tin. Bake for 1 hour 10 minutes, or until a tester comes out clean. Remove to a rack to cool. Leave the bread to cool thoroughly or partially freeze before slicing.

nutritional analysis (1 slice): calories 140; calories from fat 45; total fat 5g; saturated fat 2.5g; cholesterol 30mg; sodium 85mg; carbohydrates 23g; dietary fibre 1g; protein 2g.

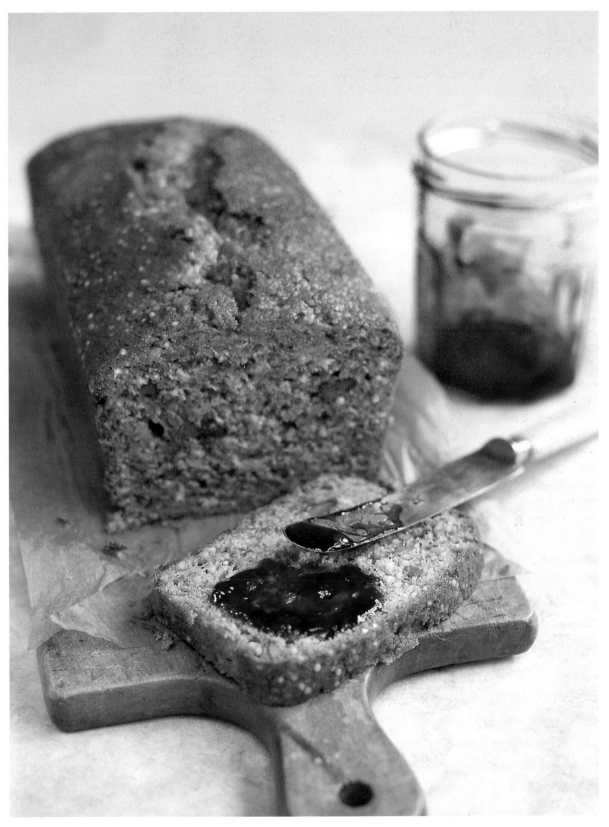

bittersweet chocolate buckwheat brownies

serves 16
makes 16 squares

ingredients

Oil cooking spray

3 x 100g (3½oz) bars high-quality plain dark chocolate

90g (3¼oz) black cherry or seedless raspberry jam

90g (3¼oz) acacia or orange blossom honey

1 large egg

2 large egg whites

1 tsp fine sea salt

Pinch of ground cinnamon (optional)

1½ tsp pure vanilla extract

70g (2½oz) buckwheat flour

45g (1½oz) coarsely chopped almonds (optional)

alternative grains

These brownies will be delicious when made with nearly any wholegrain flour.

When it comes to chocolate and health, the more bitter the better, and these brownies definitely fall into the bitter category. Go ahead, indulge yourself with these irresistible chocolate brownies with the knowledge that they are healthy, too.

1 **Preheat the oven** to 180°C (350°F, gas 4). Coat a 20cm (8in) square non-stick baking tin with oil cooking spray and set aside.

2 **Break the chocolate** into 2.5cm (1in) pieces and place in a medium-sized heatproof bowl. Gently melt the chocolate using a double boiler (or in the bowl over a saucepan of gently simmering water). Remove from the heat.

3 **In a large bowl**, combine the jam, honey, egg, egg whites, salt, cinnamon (if using), and vanilla extract. Whisk to combine thoroughly. Whisk in the flour until smooth. Slowly pour the melted chocolate into the mixture, whisking constantly. Spread the mixture in the tin. If using, sprinkle the almonds on top of the brownie mixture; pressing them slightly into the mixture.

4 **Bake for 22 minutes,** or until springy to the touch. Cool on a rack. Cut into squares when cool.

nutritional analysis (1 brownie): calories 130; calories from fat 50; total fat 6g; saturated fat 3g; cholesterol 15mg; sodium 160mg; carbohydrates 21g; dietary fibre 2g; protein 3g.

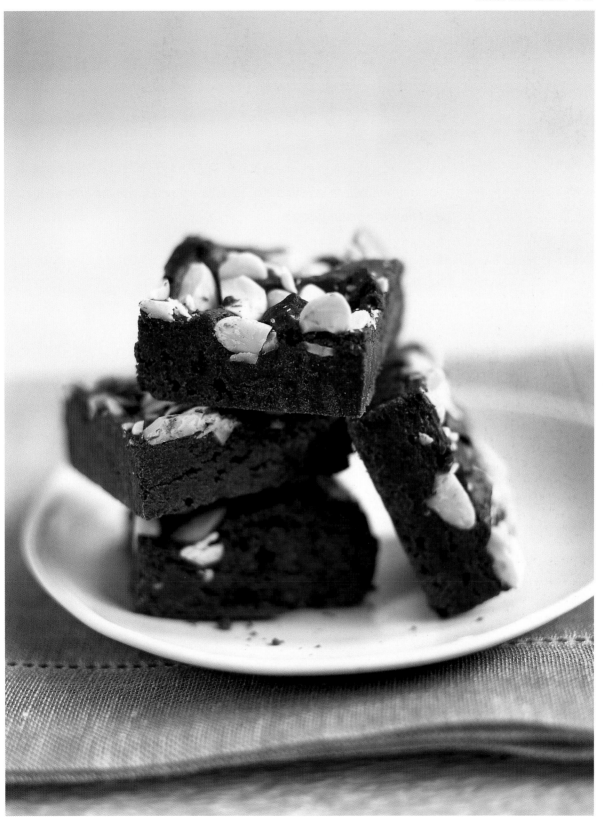

chocolate peanut butter pie

serves 10
makes 10 wedges

ingredients

1 packet instant fat-free, sugar-free chocolate pudding mix (45g/1½oz packet)

360ml (12fl oz) skimmed milk or plain soya milk

55g (2oz) rolled oats

45g (1½oz) unbleached plain flour

60g (2¼oz) light brown sugar

1 tsp cocoa powder

¼ tsp baking powder

⅛ tsp fine sea salt

4 tbsp margarine or unsalted butter, chilled and cut into pieces

125g (4½oz) unsalted smooth peanut butter

3 tbsp acacia or orange blossom honey

alternative grains

Try the crust with buckwheat or other wholegrain flour in place of plain flour for more wholegrain goodness.

The combination of chocolate and peanut butter is an all-time favourite, as they complement one another perfectly. This rich chocolate peanut butter pie unites these two flavours for a decadent, but healthy dessert.

1 **In a medium-sized bowl,** whisk the chocolate pudding mix with the milk until smooth. Chill.

2 **Preheat the oven** to 180°C (350°F, gas 4). In another large bowl, combine the oats, flour, brown sugar, cocoa, baking powder, and salt with a fork or pastry blender, breaking up any lumps. Add the margarine or butter and blend with a pastry blender or with your fingers until well combined. Press onto the bottom and sides of a 22cm (9in) non-stick pie tin.

3 **Bake for 12 minutes,** or until crisp. Remove and leave to cool on a rack.

4 **In a large bowl,** mix the peanut butter and honey together until smooth. Stir the chilled pudding into the peanut-butter mixture until smooth. Pour into the cooled pie case. Refrigerate for at least 1 hour before slicing into 10 wedges.

nutritional analysis (1 wedge): calories 230; calories from fat 100; total fat 11g; saturated fat 1.5g; cholesterol 0g; sodium 170mg; carbohydrates 26g; dietary fibre 2g; protein 6g.

brown rice pudding

serves 6

ingredients

200g (7oz) long-grain brown rice

240ml (8fl oz) fat-free evaporated milk

1 large egg

2 large egg whites

90ml (3fl oz) unsweetened apple juice

3 tbsp light brown sugar

1 tsp pure vanilla extract

45g (1½oz) raisins

1 cinnamon stick

⅛ tsp ground cinnamon

alternative grains

Prepare this comfort food with other types of rice or a rice mixture. If you can't find fat-free evaporated milk, use the regular version (but bear in mind that this has a higher fat content).

Rice pudding is a classic comfort food, but it doesn't have to be bad for you. This variation, made with brown rice and other healthy goodies, is full of flavour – and nutrition. Serve with a scoop of vanilla frozen yoghurt for a guilt-free treat.

1 **In a small saucepan** over a high heat, combine the rice with 500ml (17fl oz) water. Bring to the boil. Cover and reduce the heat to low. Simmer for 55 minutes, or until the liquid is absorbed. Remove from the heat. Leave to stand covered for 5–10 minutes.

2 **In a medium-sized saucepan,** whisk the evaporated milk, egg, egg whites, juice, brown sugar, and vanilla extract. Stir in the raisins, cinnamon stick, and warm, cooked rice. Place over a medium-low heat and cook, stirring constantly, for 8 minutes, or until thickened.

3 **Remove the cinnamon stick.** Transfer the pudding to 6 small bowls or ramekins. Cover each with greaseproof paper. Chill for at least 1 hour. Sprinkle each serving with ground cinnamon.

nutritional analysis per serving: calories 220; calories from fat 15; total fat 2g; saturated fat 0g; cholesterol 35mg; sodium 80mg; carbohydrates 42g; dietary fibre 1g; protein 8g.

BREADS AND DESSERTS

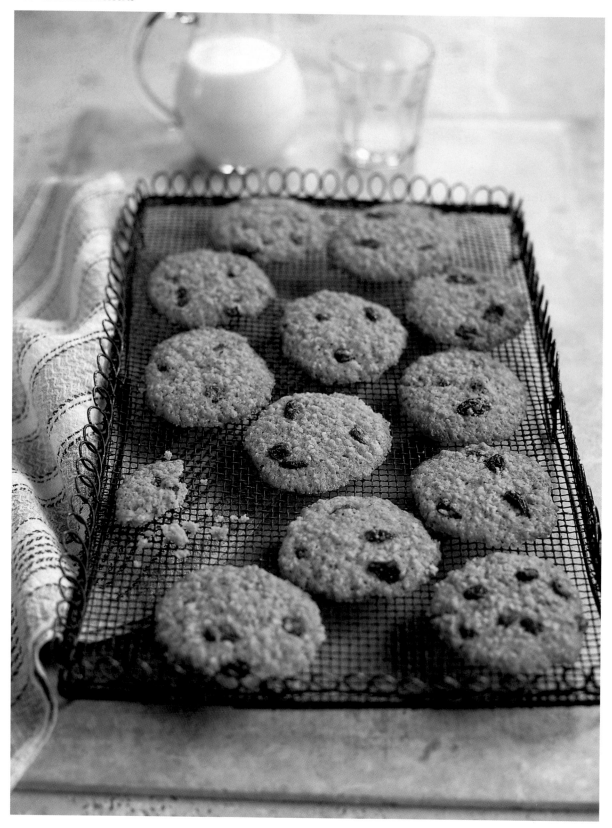

oatmeal raisin cookies

serves 12

makes 24 cookies

ingredients

8 tbsp margarine or unsalted butter, softened

100g (3½oz) granulated sugar

1 large egg

210ml (7fl oz) natural unsweetened apple sauce

½ tsp ground cinnamon

1½ tsp pure vanilla extract

100g (3½oz) unbleached plain flour

2 tbsp raw wheat germ

1 tsp bicarbonate of soda

¼ tsp fine sea salt

85g (3oz) rolled oats

55g (2oz) raisins

alternative grains

Try with a mixture of plain and granary flour of choice to increase the wholegrain benefits.

Fill your home with the heavenly aroma of these delicious cookies. They are a perfect balance of chewiness, crispness, and flavours bursting with oats, raisins, and cinnamon. And they are full of nutritional value too, providing a great source of soluble fibre.

1 **Preheat the oven** to 180°C (350°F, gas 4). In a large bowl, beat the margarine or butter and sugar until creamy with an electric mixer. Add the egg and blend well. Add the apple sauce, cinnamon, and vanilla and blend well.

2 **In a separate bowl,** combine the flour, wheat germ, bicarbonate of soda, and salt. Blend the flour mixture into the apple sauce mixture. Stir in the oats and raisins.

3 **Drop rounded tablespoons** onto baking parchment-lined or non-stick baking sheets.

4 **Bake for 12 minutes,** or until springy to the touch. Cool for 1 minute on baking sheets and remove to a rack. Cool completely.

nutrition analysis (2 cookies): calories 190; calories from fat 80; total fat 9g; saturated fat 1.5g; cholesterol 20mg; sodium 160mg; carbohydrates 26g; dietary fibre 1g; protein 3g.

pear hazelnut crisp

serves 6

ingredients

4 medium firmly ripe
Conference pears, peeled,
cored, and thinly sliced

2 tbsp light brown sugar

1 tbsp unbleached plain
flour

¼ tsp ground cinnamon

45g (1½oz) rolled oats,
uncooked

45g (1½oz) hazelnuts,
toasted, skins rubbed off
in kitchen paper, coarsely
chopped

2 tbsp light brown sugar

2 tbsp margarine or
unsalted butter, melted

⅛ tsp ground cinnamon

alternative grains

For an extra crunch, add
a sprinkle of wheat germ
to the topping mixture.

Delicious all year round, this healthy dessert works just as well with peaches and berries. Topped with fibre-rich oats and generously packed with pears, enjoy with a scoop of vanilla frozen yoghurt for a comforting treat.

1 **Preheat the oven** to 200°C (400°F, gas 6). In a large bowl, combine the pears and 3 tablespoons of water. Add the brown sugar, flour, and cinnamon and stir until the pear slices are evenly coated.

2 **Pour into a 20cm (8in)** round non-stick baking tin.

3 **To make the topping,** stir the oats, chopped hazelnuts, brown sugar, melted margarine or butter, and cinnamon in a medium-sized bowl. Continue stirring until well mixed. Sprinkle evenly over the pears.

4 **Bake for 20 minutes,** or until the pears are tender and the topping is crisp. Serve while warm. If desired, enjoy with vanilla frozen yoghurt.

nutritional analysis per serving: calories 180; calories from fat 70; total fat 7g; saturated fat 1g; cholesterol 0mg; sodium 0mg; carbohydrates 29g; dietary fibre 4g; protein 2g.

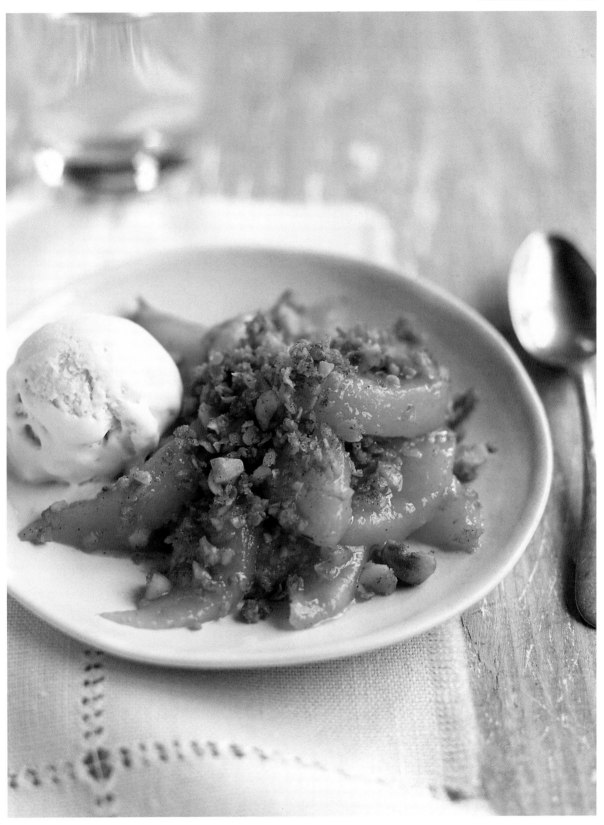

QUICK TIPS

There are a wide variety of wholegrain options available for breakfast such as porridge, wholegrain toast, and buckwheat pancakes.

•

Side dishes are a great way to boost your wholegrain intake at restaurants.

•

Ask for brown rice, rather than the usual white rice, at Chinese, Indian, Thai, and Japanese restaurants.

•

A good way of finding wholegrains when eating out is to choose the vegetarian option or dine in vegetarian restaurants.

•

Soups are another great way to sneak wholegrains into your meal.

•

Choose wholegrain breads such as wholewheat, rye, and pumpernickel instead of white bread.

eating out

Unlike foods you buy in your local supermarket, restaurant and take-away meals don't usually come with a list of ingredients, so it can be hard to know exactly what you're getting. A few strategies can help you find wholegrain choices when eating out.

1 **Start the day right**. If you enjoy going out for breakfast, take advantage of all the great wholegrain choices that are available. An excellent option is porridge – ask for skimmed milk and raisins, rather than sugar, for a delicious and filling breakfast. Other good choices include wholegrain toast, for example wholewheat or rye, wholegrain cereals, and buckwheat pancakes. Use very small amounts of butter, jams, and syrups to save calories. Remember, just because bakery products may be labelled "fat-free", this doesn't mean they are calorie-free. You still need to be careful and try to only eat small quantities.

2 **Side dishes** often provide a good way to eat more wholegrains when eating out. Restaurants are now offering a wider variety of interesting and healthy grain-based sides. Try quinoa, wild rice, brown rice, barley, and tabbouleh, which is made with bulgur wheat. Corn on the cob (as long as it is not dripping in butter) would also be a good choice.

3 **Chinese, Indian, Thai, and Japanese restaurants** are increasingly offering wholegrain options. Ask for brown rice instead of the traditional white rice. At Japanese restaurants, try buckwheat soba noodles.

4 **Vegetarian restaurants** often incorporate grains in a creative and tasty way. Even if you're not a vegetarian, consider dining in vegetarian restaurants or choosing vegetarian options when eating out.

5 **Choose soups.** These are another good way to sneak some extra grains into your meal. Look for soups that are broth-based rather than cream-based, with lots of vegetables, and wholegrains such as barley or wild rice.

6 **Choose bread wisely.** More restaurants are starting to offer a selection of wholegrain breads, such as wholewheat, rye, and pumpernickel. Instead of butter, request olive oil for dipping, which is a great source of monounsaturated ("good") fats.

eating on the run

Whether you're busy at work, travelling, or on the go at home, you don't need to give up eating healthily. With our busy lives, it is easy to turn to quick, unhealthy snacks such as chocolate or crisps. The following tips can help you to eat well when you're short of time.

1 **Don't skip breakfast.** Studies have shown that successful dieters eat breakfast. Research has also demonstrated that if you eat breakfast, you will eat less food at lunch and dinner. If you are in a rush in the morning, try one of the many wholegrain breakfast bars on offer. Prepare our Banana-walnut oat bran muffin recipe in advance (*see pp88–89*) and grab one for breakfast in the morning. For extra ease, they can be kept in the freezer at home and will defrost while you are travelling.

2 **No time for lunch?** Healthy eating is more important than ever when you're trying to keep up with a hectic schedule, as it helps your body to better withstand stress. To save time, as well as money, prepare wholegrain recipes the night before, or bring in leftovers from home and keep them in the refrigerator at the office. A great way to enjoy wholegrains at lunchtime is to add them to a sandwich such as the Quinoa tuna salad sandwich (*see p111*) or make one of our many salad recipes. About 200 grams (7oz) of cooked grains would be considered two servings of wholegrains, so for a quick option, add a few tablespoons of grains to your green salad.

3 **Be more adventurous.** More sandwich shops, cafés, and delis are offering wholegrain breads, rolls, pastas, and salad options. Look for places serving vegetarian foods or health food shops for a wider choice.

4 **Keep portions in check** when serving yourself from the salad bar or ordering sandwiches. If a whole sandwich seems too much, eat half or share with someone. Most ready-prepared salads already have dressing mixed in, so skip the added dressing to save calories.

5 **Don't be afraid to ask.** If you frequently get meals from establishments where wholegrains are not available, don't be afraid to ask them to offer these selections. These days, restaurants and eateries are becoming just as health-conscious as consumers, so it is common practice to try to meet consumer demands.

QUICK TIPS

Don't skip breakfast. Go for quick options such as wholegrain cereal bars and muffins.

•

Prepare wholegrain recipes the night before, or bring in leftovers from home, and keep in the fridge in the office.

•

Look further afield. Go to places serving vegetarian foods or health foods shops for more wholegrain options at lunchtime.

•

Watch portion sizes, especially when it is self-service. If sandwiches seem too overwhelming, eat half and save the rest for later, or share it with a friend.

•

Don't be afraid to ask your favourite sandwich shops, cafés, etc. to serve wholegrain options.

resources

Some wholegrains are easy to find but others can be a little more tricky. Consult the following list of shops and websites to help you find those less common grains, as well as organizations and associations that offer additional information on wholegrains, nutrition, and health problems.

About wholegrains

Whole Grains Council
Oldways Preservation Trust
266 Beacon Street
Boston, MA 02116 USA
www.wholegrainscouncil.org
Consortium dedicated to increasing the consumption of wholegrains and providing better health for consumers.

www.wholegrain.co.uk
Website offering practical tips and information about wholegrains.

Buying wholegrains

Fresh and Wild
69–75 Brewer Street
London W1F 9US
Tel: 020 7434 3179
Health food shop that carries a wide array of wholegrains, including quinoa, rice, amaranth, kamut, oats, rye, spelt, etc.

Planet Organic
42 Westbourne Grove
London W2 5SH
Tel: 020 7727 2227
Food shop that sells a wide variety of health foods, including wholegrains such as quinoa, rice, amaranth, kamut, oats, rye, spelt, etc.

Holland and Barrett
65 Charing Cross Road
London WC2H 0NE
Tel: 020 7287 3193
Orderline: 0870 606 6605
Email: hbcustsrv@hollandandbarrett.com
www.hollandandbarrett.com
Health food shop that carries an array of wholegrains and specialist foods.

The South African Shop
SAPRO House
Brock Lane
Maidenhead, Berks SL6 1LP
Tel: 01628 581 800
Fax: 01628 581 802
Email: mailorder@southafricanshop.co.uk
www.southafricanshop.co.uk
Shop that stocks sorghum meal. Sells items online and in their Berkshire-based shop.

Bob's Red Mill Natural Foods
5209 SE International Way
Milwaukie, OR 97222 USA
Tel: 001 800 349 2173
Fax: 001 530 653 1339
www.bobsredmill.com
US-based company that carries teff, sorghum, triticale, and other grains. Also sells a range of other wholegrain products. Ships internationally.

The Teff Company
PO Box A
Caldwell, ID 83606 USA
Tel: 001 888 822 2221
Email: info@teff.com or teffcoearthlink.net
www.teffco.com
US-based company that specializes in teff. Carries
ivory and brown varieties and ships internationally.

Other general resources
British Heart Foundation
14 Fitzhardinge Street
London W1H 6DH
Tel: 020 7935 0185
Fax: 020 7486 5820
Heart Information Line: 08450 70 80 70
Email: internet@bhf.org.uk
www.bhf.org.uk
Non-profit organization that offers information on
heart disease, as well as funding research and care.

British Nutrition Foundation
High Holborn House
52–54 High Holborn
London WC1V 6RQ
Tel: 020 7404 6504
Fax: 020 7404 6747
Email: postbox@nutrition.org.uk
www.nutrition.org.uk
Scientific and educational charity that promotes
good health by impartially interpreting and
publicizing nutritional knowledge and advice.

Coeliac UK
Suites A–D
Octagon Court
High Wycombe, Bucks HP11 2HS
Tel: 0870 444 8804
www.coeliac.co.uk
Non-profit organization offering information on
coeliac disease.

Cancerbackup
3 Bath Place
Rivington Street
London EC2A 3DR
Tel: 020 7696 9003
Fax: 020 7696 9002
Cancer Information Helpline: 0808 800 1234
www.cancerbackup.org.uk
UK charity offering information on cancer, as well
as help and support for those with the disease.

Diabetes UK
Macleod House
10 Parkway
London NW1 7AA
Tel: 020 7424 1000
Careline: 0845 120 2960
Fax: 020 7424 1001
Email: info@diabetes.org.uk
www.diabetes.org.uk
Diabetes charity that funds research and advises
on prevention and coping with the condition.

Australia and New Zealand
Macro Wholefoods
www.macrowholefoods.com.au
Organic supermarket and cafe with stores
throughout New South Wales and Victoria.
Stocks a vast range of natural, insecticide-free,
and bio-dynamic wholegrain products.

New Zealand Bio Grains Ltd
35 Dobson Street West
Ashburton 7700
Tel: 643 308 7349
Email: enquiries@BioGrains.co.nz
www.biograins.co.nz
Company that mills and supplies organic grains,
flours, pulses, and nuts. Shop online for quinoa,
barley, buckweat, rye, and other wholegrains.

index

Page numbers in **bold** refer to main entries. Main entries for grains include descriptions and types available, their history, nutritional content and health benefits, and how to cook them. Page numbers in *italics* indicate recipes, normally indexed at the main grain ingredient.

acknowledgments

authors' acknowledgments

We would like to thank the DK editorial team for helping us make the Whole Grain Diet Miracle a reality: Carl Raymond, Anja Schmidt, Shannon Beatty, Helen Murray, and Penny Warren. Also, thank you to the DK designers: Vicky Read, Anne Fisher, and Marianne Markham.

We would also like to thank the BBC, TLC, and Discovery Communications for selecting Dr Lisa Hark to host the "Honey We're Killing the Kids" show in the US.

Finally – we'd like to thank our agent, Beth Shepard, who was so excited about this project, she jumped right in to make it happen. For believing in us, listening so well, and always being there with support and encouragement, we thank you so very much.

publisher's acknowledgments

Dorling Kindersley would like to thank the following people: Kate Whitaker for the stunning photography; Luis Peral for inspired art direction; Food Stylist Sarah Tildesley, for making the recipes look great; Penny Markham for props styling; Kathy Steer for doing a superb job of Anglicizing the recipe section; and Sue Bosanko for compiling the index with a limited amount of time and space. Thanks also to wholegrains expert Cynthia Harriman for checking the accuracy of the text.

picture credits

The publisher would like to thank the following for their kind permission to reproduce their photographs: p40, Cephas Picture Library: Dario Fusaro; p56, Still Pictures: Sean Sprague; p58, Alamy Images: Stefan Auth; p59, Arco Images.

All other pictures © Dorling Kindersley. Picture researcher: Martin Copeland.

about the authors

Dr Lisa Hark is a renowned medical nutritionist with more than 20 years of experience in nutrition counselling and promoting the benefits of healthy eating in children and adults. As Director of the Nutrition Education and Prevention Programme at the University of Pennsylvania School of Medicine in Philadelphia, she is a leading nutrition educator of medical students and doctors. Dr Hark is also the co-author of DK's *Nutrition for Life*.

Dr Darwin Deen is a nationally recognized family physician who has been studying and teaching nutrition for almost 30 years. He is Professor of Family Medicine and Director of Medical Student Education at the Albert Einstein College of Medicine, where he teaches family medicine, behaviour change, and nutrition to medical students and doctors in training. Dr Deen is also co-author of DK's *Nutrition for Life* and *The Complete Guide to Nutrition in Primary Care*.

For a complete list of studies cited in this book, visit the DK website at: **www.dk.com/wholegrain**